ORTHOPEDIC CLINICS OF NORTH AMERICA

www.orthopedic.theclinics.com

Unique or Select Procedures

July 2019 • Volume 50 • Number 3

ELSEVIER

1600 John F. Kennedy Boulevard • Suite 1800 • Philadelphia, Pennsylvania, 19103-2899.

http://www.orthopedic.theclinics.com

ORTHOPEDIC CLINICS OF NORTH AMERICA Volume 50, Number 3
July 2019 ISSN 0030-5898, ISBN-13: 978-0-323-68211-4

Editor: Lauren Boyle
Developmental Editor: Kristen Helm

Orthopedic Clinics of North America (ISSN 0030-5898) is published quarterly by Elsevier Inc., 360 Park Avenue South, New York, NY 10010-1710. Months of issue are January, April, July, and October. Business and Editorial Offices: 1600 John F. Kennedy Blvd., Suite 1800, Philadelphia, PA 19103-2899. Customer Service Office: 3251 Riverport Lane, Maryland Heights, MO 63043. Periodicals postage paid at New York, NY and additional mailing offices. Subscription prices are $341.00 per year for (US individuals), $749.00 per year for (US institutions), $403.00 per year (Canadian individuals), $914.00 per year (Canadian institutions), $466.00 per year (international individuals), $914.00 per year (international institutions), $100.00 per year (US students), $220.00 per year (Canadian and international students). Foreign air speed delivery is included in all *Clinics* subscription prices. All prices are subject to change without notice. **POSTMASTER:** Send change of address to *Orthopedic Clinics of North America*, **Elsevier Health Sciences Division, Subscription Customer Service, 3251 Riverport Lane, Maryland Heights, MO 63043. Customer Service (orders, claims, online, change of address): Elsevier Health Sciences Division, Subscription Customer Service, 3251 Riverport Lane, Maryland Heights, MO 63043. Tel: 1-800-654-2452 (U.S. and Canada); 314-447-8871 (outside U.S. and Canada). Fax: 314-447-8029. E-mail:** journalscustomerservice-usa@elsevier.com **(for print support);** journalsonlinesupport-usa@elsevier.com **(for online support).**

Reprints. For copies of 100 or more, of articles in this publication, please contact the Commercial Reprints Department, Elsevier Inc., 360 Park Avenue South, New York, NY 10010-1710. Tel.: 212-633-3874; Fax: 212-633-3820; E-mail: reprints@elsevier.com.

Orthopedic Clinics of North America is covered in *MEDLINE/PubMed (Index Medicus)*, *Cinahl, Excerpta Medica*, and *Cumulative Index to Nursing and Allied Health Literature*.

EDITORIAL BOARD

CONTRIBUTORS

AUTHORS

JOSHUA ABZUG, MD
Director of Pediatric Orthopaedics and
Deputy Surgeon-in-Chief, Department of
Orthopaedics and Pediatrics, University of
Maryland School of Medicine, Timonium,
Maryland

CRAIG C. AKOH, MD
Sports Medicine Fellow, Department of
Orthopedics and Rehabilitation, University of
Wisconsin-Madison School of Medicine and
Public Health, Madison, Wisconsin

AFSHIN A. ANOUSHIRAVANI, MD
Department of Orthopaedic Surgery, Albany
Medical Center, Albany, New York

MARK E. BARATZ, MD
Clinical Professor and Vice Chairman, Director
of Hand and Upper Extremity Fellowship,
Department of Orthopaedic Surgery,
University of Pittsburgh Medical Center,
Pittsburgh, Pennsylvania

GENNADIY A. BUSEL, MD
Department of Orthopaedic Surgery, Florida
Orthopaedic Institute, Tampa, Florida

MICHELLE CAIRD, MD
Program Director, Orthopaedic Surgery,
Chief, Pediatric Orthopaedic Department,
University of Michigan, Ann Arbor, Michigan

REBECCA CHASE, DO
Philadelphia College of Osteopathic
Medicine, Philadelphia, Pennsylvania

ROBERT H. CHO, MD
Pediatric Orthopaedic Surgeon and Chief of
Staff, Orthopaedic Surgery Department,
Shriners for Children Medical Center,
Pasadena, California

ZLATAN CIZMIC, MD
Department of Orthopaedic Surgery, NYU
Langone Orthopedics, NYU Langone Health,
New York, New York

JASON L. CODDING, MD
Department of Orthopaedic Surgery, The
Everett Clinic, Everett, Washington

JEFFREY R. DUGAS, MD
Andrews Sports Medicine and Orthopaedic
Center, American Sports Medicine Institute,
Birmingham, Alabama

J. KENT ELLINGTON, MD
OrthoCarolina Foot & Ankle Institute,
Charlotte, North Carolina

JAMES E. FENG, MD
Department of Orthopaedic Surgery, NYU
Langone Orthopedics, NYU Langone Health,
New York, New York

KATHRYN FIDELER, MD
Department of Orthopaedic Surgery, Wexner
Medical Center, The Ohio State University,
Columbus, Ohio

GLENN S. FLEISIG, PhD
American Sports Medicine Institute,
Birmingham, Alabama

CORINNA C. FRANKLIN, MD
Shriners Hospitals for Children, Philadelphia,
Pennsylvania

NICHOLAS JOHN GIORI, MD, PhD
VA Palo Alto Health Care System, Palo Alto,
California; Department of Orthopaedic
Surgery, Stanford University, Stanford,
California

RACHEL Y. GOLDSTEIN, MD, MPH
Assistant Professor, Pediatric Orthopaedics,
Children's Hospital Los Angeles, Los Angeles,
California

KENNETH GRAF, MD
Cooper University Hospital, Camden, New
Jersey

KEVIN D. GRANT, MD
Department of Orthopaedic Surgery and Trauma, Beaumont Health, Royal Oak, Michigan

NADIM HALLAB, PhD
Department of Orthopedic Surgery, Rush University, Chicago, Illinois

POOYA HOSSEINZADEH, MD
Assistant Professor of Orthopaedic Surgery, Pediatric and Adolescent Orthopedic Surgery, Washington University Orthopaedics, St Louis, Missouri

JACK E. LEMONS, PhD
Department of Orthopaedic Surgery, The University of Alabama at Birmingham, Birmingham, Alabama

TRAVIS W. LITTLETON, MD
UPMC Hand and Upper Extremity Fellow, Department of Orthopaedic Surgery, University of Pittsburgh Medical Center, Pittsburgh, Pennsylvania

MARILAN LUONG, MPH
Clinical Research Coordinator, Research Department, Shriners for Children Medical Center, Pasadena, California

RANDALL DREW MADISON, MD
Trauma Fellow, Division of Orthopaedic Trauma Surgery, The University of Tennessee College of Medicine at Chattanooga/Erlanger Health System, Chattanooga, Tennessee

RAKESH MASHRU, MD
Cooper University Hospital, Camden, New Jersey

MORTEZA MEFTAH, MD
Department of Orthopaedic Surgery, NYU Langone Orthopedics, NYU Langone Health, New York, New York

WILLIAM M. MIHALKO, MD, PhD
Campbell Clinic, Department of Orthopaedic Surgery and Biomedical Engineering, The University of Tennessee Health Science Center, Memphis, Tennessee

ANDREW MILLS, MD
Department of Orthopaedic Surgery and Trauma, Beaumont Health, Royal Oak, Michigan

ARYA MINAIE, BA
Department of Orthopaedic Surgery, Washington University in St. Louis, St Louis, Missouri

HASSAN MIR, MD, MBA
Professor, Department of Orthopaedic Surgery, Director of Orthopaedic Residency Program, University of South Florida, Director of Orthopaedic Trauma Research, Florida Orthopaedic Institute, Tampa, Florida, USA

A. RYVES MOORE, MD
Andrews Sports Medicine and Orthopaedic Center, American Sports Medicine Institute, Birmingham, Alabama

PETER M. MURRAY, MD
Professor, Chair, Department of Orthopedic Surgery, Consultant, Orthopedic Surgery and Neurosurgery, Mayo Clinic, Jacksonville, Florida

DAVID NOVIKOV, BS
Department of Orthopaedic Surgery, NYU Langone Orthopedics, NYU Langone Health, New York, New York

PETER J. NOWOTARSKI, MD
Director, Division of Orthopaedic Trauma Surgery, The University of Tennessee College of Medicine at Chattanooga/Erlanger Health System, Chattanooga, Tennessee, USA

PHINIT PHISITKUL, MD
Orthopaedic Surgeon, Tri-State Specialists, LLP, Sioux City, Iowa

SELINA POON, MD
Pediatric Orthopaedic Surgeon and Director of Research, Orthopaedic Surgery Department, Shriners for Children Medical Center, Pasadena, California, USA

REY N. RAMIREZ, MD
Cooper Medical School of Rowan University, Camden, New Jersey

ZAIN SAYEED, MD, MHA
Department of Surgery, Chicago Medical School, North Chicago, Illinois

OLIVER N. SCHIPPER, MD
Anderson Orthopaedic Clinic, Arlington, Virginia

RAN SCHWARZKOPF, MD, MSc
Division of Adult Reconstructive
Surgery, Department of Orthopaedic
Surgery, NYU Langone Orthopedics,
NYU Langone Health, New York,
New York

ALISINA SHAHI, MD
Cooper University Hospital, Camden, New
Jersey

MAKSIM A. SHLYKOV, MD, MS
Orthopaedic Surgery Resident, PGY2,
Department of Orthopaedic Surgery,
Washington University in St. Louis, St Louis,
Missouri

LAURA E. STOLL, MD
Division of Orthopaedic Surgery and Sports
Medicine, Virginia Mason Medical Center,
Seattle, Washington

ROBERT J. STRAUCH, MD
Professor of Orthopedic Surgery,
NewYork-Presbyterian/Columbia University
Irving Medical Center, New York,
New York

RYAN THOMPSON, BS
Department of Surgery, Chicago
Medical School, North Chicago,
Illinois

KENNETH L. URISH, MD, PhD
Arthritis and Arthroplasty Design Group, The
Bone and Joint Center, Magee Womens
Hospital of the University of Pittsburgh
Medical Center, Departments of Orthopaedic
Surgery and Bioengineering, Clinical and
Translational Science Institute, University of
Pittsburgh, Department of Biomedical
Engineering, Carnegie Mellon University,
Pittsburgh, Pennsylvania

KUDRET USMANI, MD
Cooper University Hospital, Camden, New
Jersey

JENNIFER M. WEISS, MD
Assistant Chief of Orthopaedics, Permanente
Medical Group, Surgeon, Pediatric
Orthopaedic Department, Kaiser Permanente,
Los Angeles, California

PATRICK J. WIATER, MD
Department of Orthopaedic Surgery and
Trauma, Beaumont Health, Royal Oak,
Michigan

CHIA H. WU, MD, MBA
NewYork-Presbyterian/Columbia University
Irving Medical Center, New York, New York

JOHN C. WU, MD
Department of Orthopaedic Surgery and
Biomedical Engineering, The University of
Tennessee Campbell Clinic, Memphis,
Tennessee

CONTENTS

Knee and Hip Reconstruction
Patrick C. Toy and William M. Mihalko

> Arthrofibrosis is the pathological stiffening of a joint due to an exaggerated inflammatory response. As a relatively common complication following total knee arthroplasty (TKA), this benign appearing connective tissue hyperplasia can cause significant disability among patients as the concomitant knee pain and restricted range of motion (ROM) severely hinders postoperative rehabilitation, clinical outcomes, and basic activities of daily living (ADL). The most effective management for arthrofibrosis in the setting of TKA is prevention including preoperative patient education programs, aggressive postoperative physical therapy (PT) regimens, and anti-inflammatory medications. Operative treatments include manipulation under anesthesia, arthroscopic debridement, and quadricepsplasty.

> There has been an increased interest in the role of corrosion in total hip arthroplasty. This is based on reports of early implant failures and adverse local tissue reaction resulting from excessive corrosion at the modular interfaces of some implant designs. Orthopedic alloys are not selected based solely on their mechanical properties of strength, but rather because they possess the best balance between material properties of corrosion resistance and mechanical properties of strength. The passive layer of a metal oxide that develops on a surface of a metal serves a critical role in preventing corrosion. However, this protective layer is a dynamic structure. Aggressive corrosion occurs on implants when the kinetics of this oxide layer's destruction dominates over its generation. There is a spectrum of different types of corrosion defined by the environment and stability of the passive layer. Pitting is the localized dissolution of this protective metal oxide film. Crevice corrosion occurs with a similar mechanism but in an isolated environment that promotes corrosion. Fretting corrosion or mechanically assisted crevice corrosion (MACC) occurs with the addition of mechanical oscillating loads at the modular junction that disrupts this protective layer. Understanding this process is important to improve implant designs, surgical technique, and assessment of patients.

Trauma
John C. Weinlein and Michael J. Beebe

> Suprapatellar nailing technique is an important adjunct in the armamentarium of an orthopaedic surgeon. Although a variety of new instrumentation is required for insertion of the "suprapatellar nail", most companies now carry

these instruments. Easier positioning, maintenance of reduction, ease of intra-operative fluoroscopy, more anatomic starting trajectory, decreased malreduction rates and possible decrease in anterior knee pain are all benefits of supra-patellar nailing, thus making mastery of this technique essential for an orthopaedic surgeon.

The Reamer-Irrigator-Aspirator in Nonunion Surgery
Randall Drew Madison and Peter J. Nowotarski

The Reamer-Irrigator-Aspirator was initially designed to address the problems of fat embolism and thermal necrosis, which had previously been unsolved and have plagued clinicians since the 1940s. However, the simple addition of an inline filter and collection device allowed surgeons to efficient take advantage of the intramedullary canal as a source of autograft. RIA autograft provides large volumes of autogenous graft which have been shown to exhibit excellent osteogenic, osteoinductive, and osteoconductive properties. These features, combined with the relative ease of graft harvest and low donor site morbidity when compared to the gold standard ICBG, have made RIA autograft, at the very least, a viable alternative to ICBG. Some would suggest RIA autograft to be superior to ICBG, particularly in the setting of large segmental bone defects managed with the induced membrane technique. And although significant complications such as fracture and cortical perforation have been reported, they are preventable if proper surgical strategy and tactics are employed.

Arthroscopic-Assisted Reduction of Tibial Plateau Fractures
Rebecca Chase, Kudret Usmani, Alisina Shahi, Kenneth Graf, and Rakesh Mashru

Arthroscopic reduction of tibial plateau fractures have been gaining popularity in the orthopaedic community with advantages including accurate diagnosis and treatment of joint pathology, minimally invasive soft tissue dissection, quicker recovery of joint motion, and anatomic reduction of joint surface. The success of arthroscopic reduction depends on accurate fracture selection, with Schatzker fracture patterns I, II and III benefitting the most from effective arthroscopic assisted reduction techniques, especially when there is an intact cortical envelope or one that can be easily reduced with a clamp. With arthroscopic assisted reduction of tibial plateau fractures, patient set-up is similar to standard knee arthroscopy, but the C-arm is utilized to help with fracture reduction and fixation.

Pediatrics
Jeffrey R. Sawyer

Pediatric Orthopedic Workforce: A Review of Recent Trends
Arya Minaie, Maksim A. Shlykov, and Pooya Hosseinzadeh

Pediatric Orthopaedic Surgery has changed in many ways over the last two decades. It has changed in terms of growth, interest, demographics of surgeons, as well as in regard to new hurdles. Periodic survey of the workforce allows leadership in the field to promote healthy growth, patient safety, and address concerns as they arise. Member surveys, and recent literature confirm that there has been a sustained balance of interest and opportunity in growth of applicant numbers as well as fellowship spots. Moreover, pediatric orthopaedics has been leading the way in diversity in the realm of orthopaedics in respect to gender, and it seems as though this trend will continue into the foreseeable future. Concerns of competition are valid and appear to be rising, however case load data seems to suggest that with increased training of pediatric orthopaedists, there seems to be an adequate increase in cases. Periodic workforce analysis should continue to gauge any changes in attitudes or monitor concerns of competition.

Physician burnout is a pervasive problem affecting our workforce. Over one-third of surveyed pediatric orthopedists are experiencing symptoms of burnout. Engagement and transparency with the problem is required to support physicians throughout their career. Both personal strategies to foster resilience and systemic responses to make space for supporting physician wellness are required to truly affect change. Mindfulness is a studied tool that can be easily and strategically implemented to help combat physician burnout.

Despite the growing number of women entering medical school, female representation among orthopaedic surgery is the lowest compared to all areas of medicine. In 2014, 47.7% of students entering medical school were women, but only 13.7% of orthopedic residents were women. Pediatric orthopaedics have been successful in enrolling women compared to other orthopaedic subspecialties. The Pediatric Orthopaedic Society of North America (POSNA) is one of the largest not-for-profit professional organizations within pediatric orthopaedic surgery. This is an investigation of female representation among POSNA's membership roster providing insight into the effect on the increased gender diversity in the membership of an organization and its correlation with leadership positions at different levels within the organization.

Orthopaedic surgery remains overwhelmingly white. Comparing data from the United States Census Bureau, the Accreditation Council for Graduate Medical Education, and the American Academy of Orthopaedic Surgeons reveals that orthopaedic surgery is the least diverse of any surgical specialty, and that diversity within orthoapedics is not improving. Considerable data from both medicine and business suggests that improving diversity within our specialty would be of significant benefit to us and our patients. Multiple avenues for increasing diversity exist, from large-scale pipeline programs to personal and institutional efforts to examine our own biases and decision-making processes.

Hand and Wrist
Benjamin M. Mauck and James H. Calandruccio

Wrist denervation is a safe and effective procedure for the treatment of chronic wrist pain that can delay or eliminate the need for salvage or anatomically distorting procedure such as proximal row carpectomy. The traditional more extensive wrist denervation has evolved to procedures requiring fewer incisions. Efficacy of this procedure is corroborated by multiple publications either as a stand-alone procedure or as an adjunct to other procedures. This review provides an update on the status of wrist denervation.

Subungual melanoma is a rare form of melanoma that presents a unique set of challenges largely based on the complex anatomy of the nail unit. This form of melanoma is associated with delayed and often missed diagnosis, resulting in a high mortality risk. Longitudinal melanonychia, pigmented streaking of the nail bed, originates from the germinal matrix and affects the nail plate. It can be seen in both benign and malignant conditions. Subungual melanoma often first appears with longitudinal melanonychia. Thus, practitioners must have a high clinical suspicion in any patient with longitudinal melanonychia and a low threshold for a biopsy. The "ABCDEF" guide can be a useful tool to aid in screening any lesion of the nail bed. The authors recommend that biopsies of the nail unit be performed by a surgeon with an in depth understanding of the pathoanatomy of subungual melanoma.

Fracture fixation has evolved over the years to encompass a number of implants, including pins, screws, staples, and a variety of plate-and-screw devices. The most recent innovation in fracture fixation is shape-memory alloy (SMA) staples. Currently, SMA staples often are used as compressive fixation devices for osteotomies, arthrodesis, and fracture fixation – especially in short bones, including those of the hand and wrist. Shape-memory alloy (SMA) staples have been used successfully for osteotomies, arthrodesis, and fracture fixation, especially in small bones. SMA staples have inherent compressive properties that create a stable fracture environment that promotes primary bone healing; most effective for transverse fracture patterns. Current literature evaluating the indications for staple use, their biomechanical properties, comparison to alternative implants, and functional outcomes is limited. Understanding where SMA staple compression can be optimized and using proper indications are important factors for achieving consistent widespread success and minimizing failures. SMA staples are not a substitute for lag screw fixation or traditional plate and screw constructs, but are simply another tool that can be used for effective fracture fixation.

Shoulder and Elbow
Tyler J. Brolin

Treatment of the massive irreparable rotator cuff tear poses a challenging problem. Tendon transfers offer a solution for irreparable posterosuperior rotator cuff tears. The lower trapezius tendon transfer with incorporation of an Achilles tendon allograft has emerged as an effective way to restore strength and function in select patients. Both open and arthroscopic-assisted techniques have been described.

The anterior bundle of the ulnar collateral ligament (UCL) is the primary restraint to valgus force at the elbow, especially during the arm cocking and arm acceleration phases of the overheard throwing cycle. Injuries of the UCL can range from partial thickness tears, end avulsions, or chronic attritional ruptures with poor tissue quality. The incidence of UCL injuries is on the rise, especially among adolescent overhead athletes. If the athlete fails conservative measures, then surgery is recommended for those desiring to return to overhead sports. Over the past 40 years, UCL reconstruction has been the gold standard for all varieties of UCL injuries. Which poses the question, are some patients suitable for repair rather than reconstruction? Despite poor results with early UCL repairs, it has been shown, both biomechanically and clinically, that with proper patient selection and newer repair techniques that UCL repair can allow athletes to participate in accelerated rehabilitation and faster return to play than traditional UCL reconstruction.

Foot and Ankle

Clayton C. Bettin and Benjamin J. Grear

UNIQUE OR SELECT PROCEDURES

SERIES OF RELATED INTEREST

Clinics in Podiatric Medicine and Surgery
Clinics in Sports Medicine
Foot and Ankle Clinics
Hand Clinics
Physical Medicine and Rehabilitation Clinics of North America

PREFACE

Unique or Select Procedures

Orthopedic surgeons have always been inventors and innovators, designing and developing new techniques, better implants, and improved instruments to solve problems encountered in their patients. This issue of *Orthopedic Clinics of North America* provides insights into a number of special approaches and procedures for managing orthopedic conditions.

Thompson and colleagues remind us of the importance of recognizing the causes of and prevention of complications whenever possible. In addition to clarifying the pathophysiology of arthrofibrosis, they describe a program for preventing it after total knee arthroplasty. Trunnion corrosion in total hip arthroplasty has become a topic of much interest lately. Urish and colleagues outline the basic concepts of corrosion to help orthopedists improve implant design, surgical techniques, and patient evaluation.

Orthopedic trauma surgeons are continually developing new techniques and instrumentation to improve outcomes of fractures. Following the trend for less-invasive surgery, Usmani and colleagues describe arthroscopic-assisted reduction of tibial plateau fractures, with advantages of minimal soft tissue dissection, anatomic reduction, and quicker recovery of joint motion. An interesting addition to the fixation methods for proximal tibial fractures, the suprapatellar nail, as described by Busel and Mir, citing easier positioning, reduction maintenance, and decreased frequency of malreduction as some of the benefits. Bone grafts obtained with the reamer-irrigator-aspirator (RIA) have been shown to have excellent osteogenic, osteoinductive, and osteoconductive properties, and Madison and Nowotarski discuss the relative ease of graft harvest and low donor site morbidity, as well as the possible superior performance of RIA grafts over iliac crest bone graft in large segmental defects.

Contributors to the pediatric orthopedic section of this issue bring to light some important aspects of the subspecialty: physician burnout, racial and gender diversity, and the status of the pediatric orthopedic workforce. Goldstein and Weiss discuss the pervasive problem of physician burnout and suggest that mindfulness-based interventions are helpful to increase physical and emotional self-awareness and reduce reactivity to stressful situations. Poon and colleagues point out that, while female representation among orthopedic surgery is the lowest of all areas of medicine, pediatric orthopedics has been successful in enrolling women. Ramirez and Franklin report that orthopedic surgery is the least diverse of any surgical specialty; they suggest that improving diversity would be beneficial for surgeons and patients. A review of recent trends in the pediatric orthopedic workforce by Minaie and colleagues suggests that, although competition is increasing, there is an adequate increase in case load.

Wu and Strauch describe a less-invasive technique for wrist denervation and report its outcomes to provide an update on the status of this procedure. Subungual melanoma often is associated with delayed or missed diagnosis. Littleton and colleagues note the signs of this melanoma and present recommendations for evaluation and biopsy. Wu and colleagues discuss the advantages of nitinol (shape-memory) staples for osteotomies, arthrodesis, and fracture fixation in the hand, as well as the proper indications for their use.

Rotator cuff and ulnar collateral ligament injuries are frequent in overhead-sport athletes. Stoll and Codding describe a tendon transfer for massive irreparable rotator cuff tears, and Moore and colleagues discuss repair of the ulnar collateral ligament, highlighting patient selection and newer repair techniques.

Schipper and Ellington note that, similar to their use in the hand, nitinol staples are fast and simple to

Orthop Clin N Am 50 (2019) xv–xvi
https://doi.org/10.1016/j.ocl.2019.03.012

use in the foot, especially for midfoot and hindfoot arthrodesis. Akoh and Phisitkul discuss ligament repairs for syndesmotic injuries, including indications, techniques, outcomes, and complications.

Overall, this is a most interesting collection of diverse topics, among which every orthopedic surgeon is sure to find information relevant to and helpful in his or her practice.

Frederick M. Azar, MD
University of Tennessee–Campbell Clinic
Department of Orthopaedic Surgery
1211 Union Avenue, Suite 510
Memphis, TN 38104, USA

E-mail address:
fazar@campbellclinic.com

Knee and Hip Reconstruction

Arthrofibrosis After Total Knee Arthroplasty
Pathophysiology, Diagnosis, and Management

Ryan Thompson, BS[a,b], David Novikov, BS[a],
Zlatan Cizmic, MD[a], James E. Feng, MD[a],
Kathryn Fideler, MD[a,c], Zain Sayeed, MD, MHA[a,b],
Morteza Meftah, MD[a], Afshin A. Anoushiravani, MD[a,d],
Ran Schwarzkopf, MD, MSc[e,*]

KEYWORDS

- Total knee arthroplasty • Arthrofibrosis • Manipulation under anesthesia
- Arthroscopic debridement • Quadricepsplasty

KEY POINTS

- Arthrofibrosis is the pathologic stiffening of a joint caused by an exaggerated inflammatory response causing hyperplasia of the connective tissue around the knee.
- Arthrofibrosis following total knee arthroplasty can cause significant knee pain and restricted range of motion, severely hindering postoperative rehabilitation and basic activities of daily living.
- Disease prevention is most successful and is accomplished with preoperative patient education programs, aggressive postoperative physical therapy regimens, and anti-inflammatory medications.
- When necessary, operative techniques, including manipulation under anesthesia, arthroscopic debridement, and quadricepsplasty, can be used with varying degrees of success.

INTRODUCTION

Arthrofibrosis is the pathologic stiffening of a joint caused by an exaggerated inflammatory response. Proliferation of metaplastic fibroblasts and the excessive deposition of extracellular matrix (ECM) proteins lead to the development of thick, noncompliant, fibrous scar tissue.[1,2] As a common complication following total knee arthroplasty (TKA), this benign-appearing connective tissue hyperplasia is a cause of significant disability among patients, because the concomitant knee pain and restricted range of motion (ROM) severely hinder postoperative rehabilitation, clinical outcomes, and basic activities of daily living (ADL).[1,3,4] It is conservatively estimated that nearly 85,000 cases of arthrofibrosis occur following knee surgery in the United States per annum, with 25% of these cases requiring additional surgery in an attempt to restore adequate knee motion.[5] Moreover, for patients undergoing TKA, arthrofibrosis is estimated to be responsible for 28% of 90-day hospital

---

[a] Department of Orthopaedic Surgery, NYU Langone Orthopedics, NYU Langone Health, 301 East 17th Street, New York, NY 10003, USA; [b] Department of Surgery, Chicago Medical School, North Chicago, IL, USA; [c] Department of Orthopaedic Surgery, Wexner Medical Center, Ohio State University, Columbus, OH, USA; [d] Department of Orthopaedic Surgery, Albany Medical Center, Albany, NY, USA; [e] Division of Adult Reconstructive Surgery, Department of Orthopaedic Surgery, NYU Langone Orthopedics, NYU Langone Health, 301 East 17th Street, New York, NY 10003, USA
* Corresponding author.
E-mail address: Ran.schwarzkopf@nyumc.org

Orthop Clin N Am 50 (2019) 269–279
https://doi.org/10.1016/j.ocl.2019.02.005

readmissions and 10% of revision surgeries within the first 5 years, placing a significant burden on societal costs.[1,6] This article provides a comprehensive review of the pathophysiology of arthrofibrosis following TKA, associated risk factors, diagnostic pearls, and current management strategies in the published literature.

PATHOPHYSIOLOGY OF ARTHROFIBROSIS

Fibroblasts are the most abundant cells of the connective tissues.[1] Through their production and maintenance of the ECM's repertoire of structural, adhesive, and ground substance proteins, fibroblasts are a heterogeneous population of cells that play a major role in tissue development, architecture, and local cellular differentiation.[1,7] In the setting of tissue injury, as in TKA, fibroblasts become a vital component of scar tissue formation. In the early phases of wound healing, fibroblasts from the adjacent tissue layers produce a rich supply of collagen and adhesive proteins while providing the tractional forces needed to close the wound.[8] The tractional forces can then simulate fibroblasts to differentiate into protomyofibroblasts, upregulating the production of stress fibers.[7,8] It has been well documented that fibroblasts are also intimately linked with the inflammatory and immune response pathways, making them responsive to a wide array of inflammatory cytokines, including transforming growth factor (TGF) β1, interleukin (IL)-1β, IL-6, IL-13, IL-133, prostaglandins, and leukotrienes.[9–11] These signals induce protomyofibroblasts to undergo myofibroblastic differentiation, further promoting wound contraction and the upregulation of ECM protein production.[7–9] Concurrently, fibroblasts secrete cellular signaling factors, including reactive oxygen species, TGFβ1, IL-1β, IL-33, and CXC and CC chemokines, to promote immune cell extravasation and migration to the site of injury and inflammation. Healing of the wound is typically marked by the subsidence of inflammation and disappearance of myofibroblasts, most often through apoptosis.[7,12] However, aberrant inflammatory–wound healing interactions are thought to be the source of chronic inflammation and pathologic arthrofibrosis.[7,8,11]

DIAGNOSIS

Arthrofibrosis is diagnosed primarily on clinical assessment and ultimately confirmed with histopathologic analysis.[13] The impermeability of the joint synovium precludes the systemic circulation of potential serum-based biomarkers.

Following TKA, a low index of suspicion should be held for arthrofibrosis, particularly among patients with clinically significant loss of knee extension and/or flexion (<90° of passive flexion and <10° of full extension).[14] Although physical examination findings show substantial extension and flexion ROM deficits, the loss of knee extension is more disabling for the patients.[15] Additional findings include anterior knee pain, flexed-knee gait, quadriceps weakness, and patellofemoral painful crepitation.[16–18] Furthermore, diffuse edema, warmth, tenderness localized to the fat pad, and limited patellar mobility are characteristic findings.[16] A firm, nonfluctuant and nonedematous knee with limited patellofemoral mobility and a low-lying patella (patella baja) are also supportive findings for arthrofibrosis.[19] In contrast, a stiff knee with appropriate patellofemoral mobility typically places arthrofibrosis lower on the differential diagnosis, and may be suggestive of other disease processes, such as component malpositioning or lack of proper soft tissue balancing.[14]

Although there are no widely accepted diagnostic criteria for arthrofibrosis, there have been several attempts at defining it based on ROM deficits. Shelbourne and colleagues[19] characterized and graded arthrofibrosis into 4 categories (types 1–4) based on loss of flexion and extension ROM compared with the native contralateral knee (Table 1). More recently, Mayr and colleagues[20] defined arthrofibrosis as the presence of scar tissue in any compartment of the joint leading to restricted ROM.

Imaging

Diagnostic imaging is a useful tool in the diagnosis of arthrofibrosis.[21] Advancements in metal artifact

Table 1 Classification of arthrofibrosis based on degree of extension and flexion loss	
Type	**Extension and Flexion Deficit**
1	<10° of extension loss in the absence of flexion loss
2	>10° of extension loss in the absence of flexion loss
3	>10° of extension loss and >25° of flexion loss with a tight patella
4	>10° of extension loss, ≥30° flexion loss, and patella baja with marked patellar tightness

From Haklar U, Ayhan E, Ulku TK, et al. Arthrofibrosis of the knee. In: Doral NM, Karlsson J, editors. Sports injuries: prevention, diagnosis, treatment and rehabilitation. 2nd edition. Berlin: Springer; 2015. p. 919; with permission.

reduction sequences (MARS) for MRI can significantly reduce artifacts generated from implanted metal components, allowing physicians to assess the soft tissue within the periarticular region with high resolution.[22] In patients with stiff knees, MARS-MRI identification of nonparticulate densities of low-intensity and intraarticular adhesions within the knee are highly suggestive for arthrofibrosis.[23,24] Periarticular ultrasonography may also be a useful modality in assessing fibrotic tissue around the knee. A study performed by Boldt and colleagues[25] evaluated sonographic findings in patients with arthrofibrosis following TKA. Synovial membrane thickness was increased and the Hoffa fat pad was more pronounced; however, there were no differences among case and control cohorts with regard to the size of the joint effusion and patellar tendon thickness. The investigators concluded that synovial membrane thickening and neovascularity are unique sonographic findings that are suggestive of arthrofibrosis in the setting of TKA.[25] Radiographic examination can also identify indirect variables that may contribute to arthrofibrosis, including the use of plain film radiographs to determine joint-line elevation and computed tomography to evaluate femoral and tibial component malrotation.[14]

RISK FACTORS

There is a paucity of information evaluating patients' risk for developing arthrofibrosis, thus this article briefly summarizes the relevant risk factors, with attention to preoperative and postoperative variables predisposing TKA candidates to arthrofibrosis (Table 2).

Preoperative Risks

Several risk factors place patients at an increased risk for post-TKA stiffness, including previous knee surgery,[26] smoking,[27] diabetes mellitus,[27–29] and preoperative ROM.[30] Of these, preoperative ROM remains the most important.[30] In a study by Lizaur and colleagues,[31] patients with a preoperative flexion less than 90° had an average post-TKA flexion of 88°, significantly lower than the average 103° of flexion in patients with a preoperative flexions greater than 90°. The ability to walk, climb stairs, run, sit in a chair, and perform the most basic ADLs requires 10° to 120° of active knee flexion and is considered a tolerable ROM following TKA.[5] Accordingly, arcs of flexion less than 90° after TKA have been shown to correlate with significant patient frustration and dissatisfaction.[32]

Patient motivation and state of mind also play a critical role in patients' participation in physical

Table 2
Risk factors for development of knee arthrofibrosis following total knee arthroplasty

Perioperative Period	Risk Factor
Preoperative	Limited preoperative ROM
	History of previous knee surgeries
	Smoking
	Systemic disease (eg, diabetes)
	Patient state of mind; depression
	Genetic predisposition
Intraoperative	Inappropriate soft tissue balancing
	Component malpositioning
	Incorrect component sizing
	Excessive femoral component hyperflexion
	Excessive patellofemoral thickness
	Incorrect joint-line height
	Errors in bony resection
Postoperative	Length of immobilization
	Infection
	Complex regional pain syndrome

rehabilitation after TKA. In a study by Fisher and colleagues,[33] patients who were depressed or had a low pain tolerance were less likely to properly perform rehabilitation activities, resulting in delayed recovery and an increased likelihood of developing arthrofibrosis.

Despite limited research into the genetic factors driving arthrofibrosis, possible correlations have been found between specific human leukocyte antigen (HLA) subtypes.[2] Skutek and colleagues[2] found an association between postoperative arthrofibrosis and patients with negative HLA-Cw*07, negative DQB1*06, and positive HLA-Cw*08 haplotypes. However, these findings were performed in patients following autologous anterior cruciate ligament reconstruction, and were limited to a small sample size of 17 patients.

Surgical Risks

Iatrogenic surgical errors, such as improper soft tissue balancing, component malpositioning, and incorrect component sizing, are a common cause of postoperative stiffness following TKA.[30,34] More specifically, these surgical errors can include an inappropriately tightened posterior cruciate ligament (PCL),[35,36] excessive femoral component hyperflexion,[31] and errors in bony resection leading to so-called component overstuffing[37] and inappropriate joint-line elevation.[38,39] These surgical errors may lead to alterations in normal knee kinematics, resulting in repetitive microtrauma that is thought to trigger an inflammatory response with subsequent progression to arthrofibrosis.[39]

It is important to address methods for preventing these surgical errors in the hope of decreasing the risk for arthrofibrosis. In patients with a fixed varus deformity greater than 15°, the PCL is likely to be engaged and tight, resulting in reduced anterior tibial translation during femoral rollback, a concomitant increase in anteromedial tibial contact pressures, and a reduced flexion ark of the knee.[30,39–41] In the setting of posterior cruciate–retaining prostheses, it may be beneficial to partially release the PCL. However, caution should be exercised to not over-release the PCL because it may result in a paradoxic roll forward and anterior displacement of the femoral component, causing posterior impingement and tightening of the extensor mechanism, effectively limiting flexion.[30] Alternatively, the surgeon can opt to resect the PCL and use a posterior stabilized construct instead.

Femoral components that are placed in hyperextension or hyperflexion can limit the knee's ability to fully flex and extend, respectively.[39] To avoid excessive sagittal rotation of the femoral component, proper use of intramedullary guides or navigation systems is essential to align the femoral component with respect to the proper axis of the femur.[39,42] For axial alignment in a measured resection technique, the femoral component axis should be placed parallel to the epicondylar axis and the tibial component with the middle one-third of the tibial tubercle.[43] In the gap balancing method, femoral rotation is set parallel to the tibial cut, after the extension gap is balanced, to recreate a rectangular space, matching extension gap.[44,45]

Component overstuffing in TKA occurs when the inserted implants create a suboptimal flexion, extension, or patellofemoral space leading to reductions in the joint's arc of motion.[42] To avoid component overstuffing and inappropriate joint-line positioning, adequate tibial resections that position the joint line 1 cm proximal to the fibular head or 2 cm distal to the medial epicondyle are suggested. Furthermore, insufficient patellar resection can lead to a thick patellar bone–implant construct and cause tightness in flexion.[43] Errors in distal and posterior femoral resection can also lead to inappropriate flexion and extension gaps, further hindering postoperative knee ROM.[43] Femoral resections should be designed to restore neutral mechanical alignment with 3° to 6° valgus, and 0° to 4° of flexion.[43]

Postoperative Risks

Postoperative management is as important as proper surgical technique in preventing knee arthrofibrosis. Early motion of the knee has been hypothesized to reduce the incidence of postoperative arthrofibrosis through the breakdown of existing scar tissue, inhibition of fibrotic deposition, and adhesion formations.[46,47] It has therefore been proposed that postoperative physical therapy (PT) protocols emphasizing early motion may reduce arthrofibrosis of the knee.[39]

NONOPERATIVE MANAGEMENT

Preoperative Education

Preoperative patient education (PPE) programs are designed to improve patient adherence and outcomes through patient motivation, the encouragement of patients to take an active role in their health before and after TKA.[48] In doing so, patients are educated on proper techniques of home exercises and outpatient rehabilitation, while simultaneously setting realistic functional expectations. Patient participation is of particular value because most of these protocols include programs that demand a high degree of patient-led therapy. In a case-control study using the Danish Knee Arthroplasty Registry, PPE was associated with a decreased risk of arthrofibrosis following TKA (odds ratio, 0.16; $P = .02$).[49]

Physical Therapy

Many studies have shown clear evidence correlating decreased preoperative ROM and an increased risk for poor postoperative ROM following TKA.[29,31,50] In a randomized controlled trial (RCT) of 131 patients undergoing TKA, Beaupre and colleagues[51] evaluated the utility of a 4-week combined PPE and exercise program in improving postoperative knee ROM and function. Postoperative functional recovery was equivocal in patients who underwent this program compared with patients who did not, further disputing the effectiveness of preoperative PT.[51] It is possible that the surgery itself negates any benefits derived from preoperative PT or that the improvement in pain and function as a result of the TKA overshadow the modest improvements achieved from preoperative PT.[48,52]

Patients with arthrofibrosis after TKA pose a unique challenge to physical therapists because they require rehabilitation that focuses on restoration of ROM and the management of inflammation, pain, and swelling.[21] In the absence of arthrofibrosis, post-TKA rehabilitation tends to place more stress on building quadriceps muscle strength; however, in the setting of arthrofibrosis, it is important to prioritize targeting ROM deficits promptly because the fibrotic tissue can mature and develop resistance to exercise.[53,54] Treating ROM deficits requires a high level of patient compliance and activation, necessitating optimal pain management and an aggressive PT regimen.[55] Labraca and colleagues[56] showed that PT that began within 24 hours following TKA was associated with greater joint ROM in flexion ($16.29° \pm 11.39°$; $P = .012$) and extension ($2.12° \pm 3.19°$; $P = .035$). Although PT should be aggressive to achieve optimal ROM, it is important to avoid an overly aggressive protocol because it can precipitate an inflammatory reaction that can worsen pain and further joint contracture or cause patella fracture or tendon rupture.[39]

The use of continuous passive motion (CPM) machines has been a debated topic regarding the prevention of knee stiffness following TKA because there has been inconclusive evidence of its ability to improve ROM and reduce the need for manipulation under anesthesia (MUA).[57] In a Cochrane Review of 24 RCTs with a cumulative 1445 TKA patients, CPM enacted only a modest difference in active knee flexion.[58] The gain in ROM was clinically insignificant because the mean active ROM in patients without CPM was 78° compared with 80° in patients using CPM machines. In addition, Boese and colleagues[57] conducted a 160-patient RCT evaluating the ability of CPM devices to improve postoperative ROM. The investigators compared outcomes among a group of patients who received a CPM device moving from 0° to 110°, a group of patients who received a CPM device that was fixed at 90° in flexion, and a group of patients who did not receive a CPM device.[57] There was no difference found between the 3 groups with regard to postoperative ROM, further disputing the benefit of using CPM in TKA patients to improve knee ROM.[57]

In cases in which PT fails to improve arthrofibrosis, noninvasive assistive devices, such as various knee orthotics, have shown promise.[59–61] The hinged metal brace uses the principle of static progressive stretching, a technique that holds the joint at a position near the end of ROM followed by incremental increases in displacement between the thigh and leg over time.[59] Bonutti and colleagues[59] reported on outcomes in 25 patients who were refractory to PT and were treated with this device. After a median treatment interval of 7 weeks, the investigators showed a median 25° (range, 8°–82°) increase in ROM, median 19° (range, 5°–80°) increase in knee active flexion, and 92% satisfaction in results among the patients.[59]

Antiinflammatories and Other Medications

Although the exact cause of arthrofibrosis is poorly understood, a strong relationship with inflammatory markers, postoperative pain, and pain during rehabilitation has been observed.[9–11,62,63] Multiple studies have correlated increased perioperative pain with arthrofibrosis and decreased ROM in total joint arthroplasty patients.[64–67] Therefore, a multimodal approach to decreasing inflammation and controlling pain can improve patient mobilization and prevent arthrofibrosis.

Nonsteroidal anti-inflammatory drugs (NSAIDs) inhibit 2 of the most common inflammatory pathways, cyclooxygenase (COX)-1 and COX-2, effectively decreasing prostaglandin synthesis. Although, prostaglandins do not directly mediate pain, they perpetuate the inflammatory cycle and increase the excitability of nociceptors in injured tissues.[68] Feng and colleagues[69] noted significantly decreased levels of regional cytokines and leukocytes in knee drainage fluid from patients who received a preoperative dose of rofecoxib (a selective COX-2 inhibitor) compared with a placebo. In the control group, the total number of leukocytes increased approximately 2 to 4 times above the baseline, starting 2 hours after TKA, and continuing for 48 hours.[69] However, patients who received 25 mg of rofecoxib before surgery only showed a 2-fold increase in leukocytes. The measured levels of IL-6 and tumor necrosis factor alpha were also significantly lower in joint fluid by 50% to 60% up to 48 hours. Patients using rofecoxib showed improved pain scores at rest and with activity. At rest, the mean modified numerical pain rating scales were significantly lower in the rofecoxib group at 24 hours (0.3 ± 0.1 vs 0.9 ± 0.1; $P<.05$) and at 48 hours (0.1 ± 0.1 vs 0.7 ± 0.1; $P<.05$) following surgery.

A similar outcome was noted when patients were active in the rofecoxib group with lower pain scores at 24 hours (0.8 ± 0.5 vs 1.8 ± 1.2; $P<.05$) and 48 hours (0.7 ± 0.4 vs 1.6 ± 1.0; $P<.005$) following surgery.[69] Buvanendran and colleagues[70] found that patients who received postoperative rofecoxib were able to achieve higher joint ROM with shorter time in PT after TKA. A significant increase in both active (84.2° vs 73.2°; $P = .03$) and passive knee flexion (90.5° vs 81.8°; $P = .05$) was noted as early as discharge compared with the placebo group. Furthermore, mean flexion continued to be significantly superior in the patients receiving rofecoxib at 1 month postoperatively (109.3° vs 100.8°; $P = .01$). As such, perioperative NSAID use may reduce inflammation, minimize the pathogenesis of fibrotic scar formation, and decrease pain in the early rehabilitation phase, allowing more aggressive physiotherapy regimens following TKA.

In an effort rehabilitate TKA recipients, an emphasis has been placed on narcotic-sparing pain protocols, which include NSAIDs, acetaminophen, peripheral nerve blocks, long-lasting local anesthetics, periarticular infiltration, epidural infusions, oral and intravenous opioids, steroids, and anticonvulsants.[71–73] Lavernia and colleagues[66] retrospectively examined the effects of a multimodal pain management protocol, consisting of PPE, perioperative pain cocktails, femoral nerve blocks, and intraoperative analgesic injections, on outcomes following TKA. The investigators showed a reduced incidence of MUA from 4.75% (37 out of 778) to 2.24% (8 out of 357) compared with the traditional pain protocol, comprising patient-controlled analgesia pumps and opioid medications.[66] Ranawat and colleagues[74] described improved outcomes with their perioperative pain protocol for TKA patients. Using a multimodal protocol, Ranawat and colleagues[74] reported improved recovery and a minimum of 90° ROM with more than 85% of patients reporting 110° ROM. Furthermore, patients had higher rates of ambulation (98% vs 80%) and quicker recovery in PT starting on postoperative day 1. More recently, they have used a combination of epidural infusions and femoral nerve blocks with or without intravenous pain-control analgesia, as well as a transition from general to regional anesthesia. In the evolving Bundled Payments for Care Improvement environment, an increased use of pain services and a multidisciplinary team care approach has emerged as an important part of proper pain management following TKA.[65]

Supplemental cryotherapy is sometimes suggested in an effort to reduce swelling and inflammation.[75] It is a treatment that uses cold compression in the postoperative period and is thought to help with pain management, ROM, and knee function. In a recent RCT by Kullenberg and colleagues,[76] 86 patients were randomized to receive either cryotherapy or no treatment following TKA. The investigators showed that patients who received cryotherapy in the immediate postoperative period showed improved ROM measurements 3 weeks following TKA (98.9 vs 87.6; $P = .0045$), further underscoring its potential utility.

OPERATIVE MANAGEMENT
Manipulation Under Anesthesia
For TKA patients that fail PT and continue to experience functionally limiting knee flexion, MUA is the first-line operative treatment of choice.[77,78] Performed in the operating room, patients are placed under conscious sedation and maximal muscle relaxation is obtained.[77,79] The ipsilateral hip is subsequently flexed to 90° while the surgeon grasps the proximal third of the tibia and the knee is flexed slowly until audible and palpable separation of adhesions no longer occur. Use of the distal third of the tibia should be avoided to prevent excessive leverage on the joint and potential supracondylar fractures.[79]

In a prospective cohort study by Esler and colleagues,[80] patients who consented to MUA showed an average gain in active knee flexion of 33° that was sustained from 6 weeks to 1 year. In contrast, those who declined were only able to recover 3.1° of knee flexion ($P = .23$).[80] These findings are congruent with more recent studies and systematic reviews, which have reported a 30° to 47° recovery of knee flexion following MUA.[77,78,81] However, current indications for MUA vary between studies, with cutoffs ranging widely between 80° and 110°, potentially concealing the true ROM gained following MUA.[77,80] Clinically, patients should be evaluated on a case-by-case basis for functional limitations secondary to subjective stiffness and restricted knee ROM. Patient background, culture, and religion should also be accounted for because these factors may involve kneeling or cross-legged sitting, requiring deeper knee flexion angles. Although the risks and benefits of increased ROM should also be weighed against potential complications, such as supracondylar fractures and patellar tendon ruptures, their incidences have been inadequately reported in the literature.[81–83]

MUA timing also plays a critical role in the extent of knee flexion regained.[77,84] In a retrospective study by Issa and colleagues,[77] patients who had received MUA within a 12-week window after surgery showed a significantly higher recovery of knee flexion (36.5° vs 17°; $P<.0001$) and Knee Society objective (89 vs 84 points; $P<.05$) and function (88 vs 83 points; $P<.045$) scores than those after 12 weeks.[77] Subset analysis of these groups showed worsening outcomes for MUAs between 13 to 26 weeks versus greater than 26 weeks (21° vs 12°; $P<.01$), but no significant differences between 0 to 6 weeks versus 6 to 12 weeks following surgery (36° vs 38°; $P<.89$). In summary, despite the lack of high-quality RCTs comparing the outcomes of MUA with non-MUA intervention, the current orthopedic literature strongly supports MUA as an effective first-line intervention in the setting of unsatisfactory knee flexion and function, and should ideally be performed within 12 weeks of surgery (Fig. 1).[77,78,80] For patients with ongoing infection, component malalignment, or an elevated joint-line, MUA is contraindicated and the patient should instead be evaluated for revision TKA to address the primary underlying condition.[77]

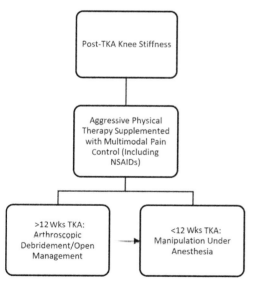

Fig. 1. Intervention protocol for TKA candidates. Patients with knee stiffness should be immediately started on an aggressive physical therapy regimen, supplemented with a multimodal pain control that includes NSAID therapy. Treatment failure should progress to more aggressive management. For patients within 12 weeks of TKA, manipulation under anesthesia should be pursued. Patients failing manipulation, or who are outside the 12-week window, should progress to arthroscopic debridement and/or possible open management.

Arthroscopic Lysis of Adhesions

The formation of adhesions in the arthrofibrotic knee occurs primarily between the capsule and femoral condyles, as well as in the anterior interval, infrapatellar fat pad, and pretibial recess.[85] Arthroscopic lysis of adhesions (LOA) is therefore a minimally invasive surgical approach that allows for direct visualization and treatment of the focal and diffuse pathologic fibrous scar tissue using motorized shaver instruments and radiofrequency ablation devices.[85]

Although there are few studies examining the outcomes of arthroscopic LOA, retrospective studies report good outcomes. A retrospective study by Schwarzkopf and colleagues[86] reported a significant gain of 23.75° of total ROM following arthroscopic LOA with MUA. Higher preoperative WOMAC (Western Ontario and McMaster Universities) scores, shorter patients, and body mass index greater than 30 kg/m^2 were also correlated with greater ROM gains. Several other studies have also shown similar gains ranging from 18.5° to 60° of total ROM.[78,87]

Although posterior capsular adhesions are thought to be the primary contributor of flexion contractures, and access to this region of the knee is arthroscopically limited, previous studies have been reassuring. In a retrospective study of arthroscopic LOA after failed MUA by Tjoumakaris and colleagues,[87] the average extension deficit was significantly decreased from 16° to 4° at final follow-up (minimum 12 months, average 31 months) despite no attempt at posterior release in of any patients in the cohort. Furthermore, in a separate retrospective study of 18 patients with posterior stabilized TKAs, arthroscopic LOA again showed significant reductions in extension deficits, from 9.17° to 3.06°.[88] In addition, unlike MUA alone, the timing of arthroscopy does not seem to affect outcomes, and successful results have been reported up to 1 year following TKA.[78]

Open Scar Excision and Revision Knee Arthroplasty

In a small number of patients, extensive periarticular and intraarticular fibrosis makes it very difficult to use arthroscopic treatments. These refractory cases necessitate an open scar excision with debridement and soft tissue release for better visualization and easier access to the fibrotic tissue.[89] A retrospective study by Millett and colleagues[89] reported improvements in 8 knees, with gains of flexion from 81° to 125° and reductions in extension loss from 18.8° to 1.25°. In addition, Lysholm II scores improved by 35.5 points per patient and all patients were satisfied with their outcomes.[89]

Once all other treatment options are exhausted or if there is clear evidence of implant malposition, revision TKA should be considered. Outcomes following revision TKA for arthrofibrosis have been modest compared with those following revision TKA for other causes, such as instability or loosening.[90] Kim and colleagues reported improvements in mean Knee Society function scores (40–58 points), mean Knee Society pain scores (15–47 points), and mean knee ROM (55° to 82°) among 52 patients that underwent revision TKA for arthrofibrosis.

SUMMARY

Arthrofibrosis is a common complication following TKA, causing patients significant functional disability. The emergence of rapid rehabilitation protocols and perioperative NSAIDs has reduced the prevalence of arthrofibrosis following TKA. An understanding of the pathophysiologic underpinnings, associated risk factors, and management strategies can aid in the treatment of these patients.

REFERENCES

1. Abdul N, Dixon D, Walker A, et al. Fibrosis is a common outcome following total knee arthroplasty. Sci Rep 2015;5:16469.

2. Skutek M, Elsner H-A, Slateva K, et al. Screening for arthrofibrosis after anterior cruciate ligament reconstruction: analysis of association with human leukocyte antigen. Arthroscopy 2004;20(5):469–73.

3. Dixon D, Coates J, Del Carpio Pons A, et al. A potential mode of action for Anakinra in patients with arthrofibrosis following total knee arthroplasty. Sci Rep 2015;5:16466.

4. Faust I, Traut P, Nolting F, et al. Human xylosyltransferases - mediators of arthrofibrosis? New pathomechanistic insights into arthrofibrotic remodeling after knee replacement therapy. Sci Rep 2015;5:12537.

5. Stephenson JJ, Quimbo RA, Gu T. Knee-attributable medical costs and risk of re-surgery among patients utilizing non-surgical treatment options for knee arthrofibrosis in a managed care population. Curr Med Res Opin 2010; 26(5):1109–18.

6. Schroer WC, Berend KR, Lombardi AV, et al. Why are total knees failing today? Etiology of total knee revision in 2010 and 2011. J Arthroplasty 2013;28(8 Suppl):116–9.

7. Li B, Wang JH-C. Fibroblasts and myofibroblasts in wound healing: force generation and measurement. J Tissue Viability 2011;20(4):108–20.

8. Tomasek JJ, Gabbiani G, Hinz B, et al. Outcomes and predictors of success for arthroscopic lysis of adhesions for the stiff total knee arthroplasty. Nat Rev Mol Cell Biol 2002;3(5):349–63.

9. Kendall RT, Feghali-Bostwick CA. Fibroblasts in fibrosis: novel roles and mediators. Front Pharmacol 2014;5:123.

10. Buckley CD, Pilling D, Lord JM, et al. Fibroblasts regulate the switch from acute resolving to chronic persistent inflammation. Trends Immunol 2001; 22(4):199–204.

11. Border WA, Noble NA. Transforming growth factor β in tissue fibrosis. N Engl J Med 1994;331(19): 1286–92.

12. Van Linthout S, Miteva K, Tschope C. Crosstalk between fibroblast and inflammatory cells. Cardiovasc Res 2014;102(2):258–69.

13. Krenn V, Ruppert M, Knöß P, et al. Synovialitis vom arthrofibrotischen Typ. Z Rheumatol 2013;72(3): 270–8.

14. Maloney WJ. The stiff total knee arthroplasty: evaluation and management. J Arthroplasty 2002;17(4 Suppl 1):71–3. Available at: http://www.ncbi.nlm. nih.gov/pubmed/12068410. Accessed February 2, 2018.

15. Lindenfeld TN, Wojtys EM, Arbor A, et al. Operative Treatment of Arthrofibrosis of the Knee* [dagger]. J Bone Jt Surg 1999;81(12):1772–84. Available at: https://ovidsp.tx.ovid.com/sp-3.28. 0a/ovidweb.cgi?QS2=434f4e1a73d37e8cf5d3d7f4c 06fe8b477edbc64438c728ea13b4923903f76c05e97 6e222cbf5ff8a3af52bce32f92d9bfbb52925f8689b13 d90a6f6b1159b16a6a1de9fbe3b147bb312064445a 9276f4d590db43682b9ed4d64bc6fa4d42f9c4af71 f547. Accessed April 12, 2018.

16. Noyes FR, Barber-Westin SD. Noyes' knee disorders : surgery, rehabilitation, clinical outcomes.

17. Haklar U, Ayhan E, Ulku TK, et al. Arthrofibrosis of the knee. In: Sports injuries. Berlin: Springer Berlin Heidelberg; 2015. p. 915–31. https://doi.org/10. 1007/978-3-642-36569-0_100.

18. Sachs RA, Daniel DM, Stone ML, et al. Patellofemoral problems after anterior cruciate ligament reconstruction. Am J Sports Med 1989;17(6):760–5.

19. Shelbourne KD, Patel DV, Martini DJ. Classification and management of arthrofibrosis of the knee after anterior cruciate ligament reconstruction. Am J Sports Med 1996;24(6):857–62.

20. Mayr HO, Weig TG, Plitz W. Arthrofibrosis following ACL reconstruction—reasons and outcome. Arch Orthop Trauma Surg 2004;124(8):518–22.

21. Cheuy VA, Foran JRH, Paxton RJ, et al. Arthrofibrosis associated with total knee arthroplasty. J Arthroplasty 2017;32(8):2604–11.

22. Heyse TJ, Chong LR, Davis J, et al. MRI analysis of the component-bone interface after TKA. Knee 2012;19(4):290–4.

23. Potter HG, Foo LF. Magnetic resonance imaging of joint arthroplasty. Orthop Clin North Am 2006; 37(3):361–73. vi-vii.

24. Shang P, Liu HX, Zhang Y, et al. A mini-invasive technique for severe arthrofibrosis of the knee: A technical note. Injury 2016;47(8):1867–70.

25. Boldt JG, Munzinger UK, Zanetti M, et al. Arthrofibrosis associated with total knee arthroplasty: gray-scale and power Doppler sonographic findings. AJR Am J Roentgenol 2004;182(2):337–40.

26. Scranton PE. Management of knee pain and stiffness after total knee arthroplasty. J Arthroplasty 2001;16(4):428–35.

27. Jordan L, Kligman M, Sculco TP. Total knee arthroplasty in patients with poliomyelitis. J Arthroplasty 2007;22(4):543–8.

28. Meding JB, Reddleman K, Keating ME, et al. Total knee replacement in patients with diabetes mellitus. Clin Orthop Relat Res 2003;416(416):208–16.

29. Gandhi R, de Beer J, Leone J, et al. Predictive risk factors for stiff knees in total knee arthroplasty. J Arthroplasty 2006;21(1):46–52.

30. Scuderi GR. The stiff total knee arthroplasty. Knee 2005;20(4):23–6.

31. Lizaur A, Marco L, Cebrian R. Preoperative factors influencing the range of movement after total knee arthroplasty for severe osteoarthritis. J Bone Joint Surg Br 1997;79(4):626–9.

32. Lam LO, Swift S, Shakespeare D. Fixed flexion deformity and flexion after knee arthroplasty. What happens in the first 12 months after surgery and can a poor outcome be predicted? Knee 2003;10(2):181–5.

33. Fisher DA, Dierckman B, Watts MR, et al. Looks good but feels bad: factors that contribute to poor results after total knee arthroplasty. J Arthroplasty 2007;22(6 SUPPL):39–42.

34. Christensen CP, Crawford JJ, Olin MD, et al. Revision of the stiff total knee arthroplasty. J Arthroplasty 2002;17(4):409–15.

35. Insall JN, Hood RW, Flawn LB, et al. The total condylar knee prosthesis in gonarthrosis. A five to nine-year follow-up of the first one hundred consecutive replacements. J Bone Joint Surg Am 1983;65(5):619–28.

36. Ranawat CS, Boachie-Adjei O. Survivorship analysis and results of total condylar knee arthroplasty. Eight- to 11-year follow-up period. Clin Orthop Relat Res 1988;(226):6–13.

37. Callahan CM. Patient outcomes following tricompartmental total knee replacement. JAMA 1994; 271(17):1349.

38. Maloney W, Schurman D. The effects of implant design on range of motion after total knee arthroplasty: total condylar versus posterior stabilized total condylar designs. Clin Orthop Relat Res 1992; 278(278):147–51.

39. Schiavone Panni A, Cerciello S, Vasso M, et al. Stiffness in total knee arthroplasty. J Orthop Traumatol 2009;10(3):111–8.

40. Lombardi AV, Mallory TH, Fada RA, et al. An algorithm for the posterior cruciate ligament in total knee arthroplasty. Clin Orthop Relat Res 2001;392: 75–87. Available at: http://www.ncbi.nlm.nih.gov/pubmed/11716428. Accessed February 2, 2018.

41. Laskin RS. The Insall Award. Total knee replacement with posterior cruciate ligament retention in patients with a fixed varus deformity. Clin Orthop Relat Res 1996;331:29–34.

42. Laskin RS, Beksac B. Stiffness after total knee arthroplasty. J Arthroplasty 2004;19(4):41–6.

43. Su EP, Su SL, Della Valle AG. Stiffness after TKR: how to avoid repeat surgery. Orthopedics 2010; 33(9):658.

44. Meftah M, Blum YC, Raja D, et al. Correcting fixed varus deformity with flexion contracture during total knee arthroplasty: the "inside-out" technique. AAOS exhibit selection. J Bone Joint Surg Am 2012;94(10):e66.

45. Meftah M, Ranawat AS, Ranawat CS. Ten-year follow-up of a rotating-platform, posterior-stabilized total knee arthroplasty. J Bone Joint Surg Am 2012;94(5):426–32.

46. O'Driscoll SW, Keeley FW, Salter RB. Durability of regenerated articular cartilage produced by free autogenous periosteal grafts in major full-thickness defects in joint surfaces under the influence of continuous passive motion. A follow-up report at one year. J Bone Joint Surg Am 1988;70(4):595–606.

47. Delaney JP, O'Driscoll SW, Salter RB. Neochondrogenesis in free intraarticular periosteal autografts in an immobilized and paralyzed limb. An experimental investigation in the rabbit. Clin Orthop Relat Res 1989;248:278–82.

48. Wallis JA, Taylor NF. Pre-operative interventions (non-surgical and non-pharmacological) for patients with hip or knee osteoarthritis awaiting joint replacement surgery - a systematic review and meta-analysis. Osteoarthr Cartil 2011;19(12): 1381–95.

49. Livbjerg AE, Froekjaer S, Simonsen O, et al. Preoperative patient education is associated with decreased risk of arthrofibrosis after total knee arthroplasty. J Arthroplasty 2013;28(8):1282–5.

50. Ritter MA, Stringer EA. Predictive range of motion after total knee replacement. Clin Orthop Relat Res 1979;143:115–9. Available at: https://insights.ovid.com/crossref?an=00003086-197909000-00016. Accessed March 19, 2018.

51. Beaupre LA, Lier D, Davies DM, et al. The effect of a preoperative exercise and education program on functional recovery, health related quality of life, and health service utilization following primary total knee arthroplasty. J Rheumatol 2004;31(6):1166–73.

52. D'Lima DD, Colwell CW, Morris BA, et al. The effect of preoperative exercise on total knee replacement outcomes. Clin Orthop Relat Res 1996;326:174–82.

53. Kalson NS, Borthwick LA, Mann DA, et al. International consensus on the definition and classification of fibrosis of the knee joint. Bone Joint J 2016;98-B(11):1479–88.

54. Magit D, Wolff A, Sutton K, et al. Arthrofibrosis of the knee. J Am Acad Orthop Surg 2007;15(11):682–94.

55. Ranawat CS, Ranawat AS, Mehta A. Total knee arthroplasty rehabilitation protocol: what makes the difference? J Arthroplasty 2003;18(3 Suppl 1):27–30.

56. Labraca NS, Castro-Sánchez AM, Matarán-Peñarrocha GA, et al. Benefits of starting rehabilitation within 24 hours of primary total knee arthroplasty: randomized clinical trial. Clin Rehabil 2011;25(6):557–66.

57. Boese CK, Weis M, Phillips T, et al. The efficacy of continuous passive motion after total knee arthroplasty: a comparison of three protocols. J Arthroplasty 2014;29(6):1158–62.

58. Harvey LA, Brosseau L, Herbert RD. Continuous passive motion following total knee arthroplasty in people with arthritis. Cochrane Database Syst Rev 2010;(3):CD004260.

59. Bonutti PM, Marulanda GA, McGrath MS, et al. Static progressive stretch improves range of motion in arthrofibrosis following total knee arthroplasty. Knee Surg Sports Traumatol Arthrosc 2010;18(2):194–9.

60. Seyler TM, Marker DR, Bhave A, et al. Functional problems and arthrofibrosis following total knee arthroplasty. J Bone Joint Surg Am 2007;89:59–69.

61. McElroy MJ, Johnson AJ, Zywiel MG, et al. Devices for the prevention and treatment of knee stiffness after total knee arthroplasty. Expert Rev Med Devices 2011;8(1):57–65.

62. Bosch U, Zeichen J, Lobenhoffer P, et al. Arthrofibrose Ein chronischer inflammatorischer Proze? Arthroskopie 1999;3(12):117–20.

63. Bosch U, Zeichen J, Skutek M, et al. Arthrofibrosis is the result of a T cell mediated immune response. Knee Surg Sports Traumatol Arthrosc 2001;9(5):282–9.

64. Ryu J, Saito S, Yamamoto K, et al. Factors influencing the postoperative range of motion in total knee arthroplasty. Bull Hosp Jt Dis 1993;53(3):35–40.

65. Maheshwari AV, Blum YC, Shekhar L, et al. Multimodal pain management after total hip and knee arthroplasty at the Ranawat Orthopaedic Center. Clin Orthop Relat Res 2009;467(6):1418–23.

66. Lavernia C, Cardona D, Rossi MD, et al. Multimodal pain management and arthrofibrosis. J Arthroplasty 2008;23(6 Suppl 1):74–9.

67. Brander VA, Stulberg SD, Adams AD, et al. Ranawat award paper: predicting total knee replacement pain. Clin Orthop Relat Res 2003;416:27–36.

68. Steinmeyer J. Pharmacological basis for the therapy of pain and inflammation with nonsteroidal anti-inflammatory drugs. Arthritis Res 2000;2(5):379–85.

69. Feng Y, Ju H, Yang B, et al. Effects of a selective cyclooxygenase-2 inhibitor on postoperative inflammatory reaction and pain after total knee replacement. J Pain 2008;9(1):45–52.

70. Buvanendran A, Kroin JS, Tuman KJ, et al. Effects of perioperative administration of a selective cyclooxygenase 2 inhibitor on pain management and recovery of function after knee replacement. JAMA 2003;290(18):2411.

71. Halawi MJ, Grant SA, Bolognesi MP. Multimodal analgesia for total joint arthroplasty. Orthopedics 2015;38(7):e616–25.

72. Parvizi J, Bloomfield MR. Multimodal pain management in orthopedics: implications for joint arthroplasty surgery. Orthopedics 2013;36(2):7–14.

73. Lavernia CJ, Alcerro JC, Contreras JS. Knee arthroplasty: growing trends and future problems. Int J Clin Rheumtol 2010;5(5):565–79.

74. Ranawat CS, Ranawat AS, Parvataneni HK. How I manage pain after total knee replacement. Semin Arthroplasty 2008;19(3):237–42.

75. Eakin CL. Knee arthrofibrosis: prevention and management of a potentially devastating condition. Phys Sportsmed 2001;29(3):31–42.

76. Kullenberg B, Ylipaa S, Soderlund K, et al. Postoperative cryotherapy after total knee arthroplasty: a prospective study of 86 patients. J Arthroplasty 2006;21(8):1175–9.

77. Issa K, Banerjee S, Kester MA, et al. The effect of timing of manipulation under anesthesia to improve range of motion and functional outcomes following total knee arthroplasty. J Bone Jt Surg 2014;96(16):1349–57.

78. Fitzsimmons SE, Vazquez EA, Bronson MJ. How to treat the stiff total knee arthroplasty?: a systematic review. Clin Orthop Relat Res 2010;468(4):1096–106.

79. Fox JL, Poss R. The role of manipulation following total knee replacement. J Bone Joint Surg Am 1981;63(3):357–62.

80. Esler CNN, Lock K, Harper WMM, et al. Manipulation of total knee replacements. Is the flexion gained retained? J Bone Joint Surg Br 1999;81(1):27–9.

81. Yeoh D, Nicolaou N, Goddard R, et al. Manipulation under anaesthesia post total knee replacement: long term follow up. Knee 2012;19(4):329–31.

82. Ipach I, Mittag F, Lahrmann J, et al. Arthrofibrosis after TKA - influence factors on the absolute flexion

and gain in flexion after manipulation under anaesthesia. BMC Musculoskelet Disord 2011;12:184.

83. Mohammed R, Syed S, Ahmed N. Manipulation under anaesthesia for stiffness following knee arthroplasty. Ann R Coll Surg Engl 2009;91(3):220–3.

84. Mamarelis G, Sunil-Kumar KH, Khanduja V. Timing of manipulation under anaesthesia for stiffness after total knee arthroplasty. Ann Transl Med 2015; 3(20):316.

85. Enad JG. Arthroscopic lysis of adhesions for the stiff total knee arthroplasty. Arthrosc Tech 2014; 3(5):e611–4.

86. Schwarzkopf R, William A, Deering RM, et al. Arthroscopic lysis of adhesions for stiff total knee arthroplasty. Orthopedics 2013;36(12): e1544–8.

87. Tjoumakaris FP, Tucker BC, Post Z, et al. Arthroscopic lysis of adhesions for the stiff total knee: results after failed manipulation. Orthopedics 2014; 37(5):e482–7.

88. Bodendorfer BM, Kotler JA, Zelenty WD, et al. Outcomes and predictors of success for arthroscopic lysis of adhesions for the stiff total knee arthroplasty. Orthopedics 2017;40(6):e1062–8.

89. Millett PJ, Williams RJ, Wickiewicz TL. Open debridement and soft tissue release as a salvage procedure for the severely arthrofibrotic knee. Am J Sports Med 1999;27(5):552–61.

90. Pun SY, Ries MD. Effect of gender and preoperative diagnosis on results of revision total knee arthroplasty. Clin Orthop Relat Res 2008;466:2701–5. Springer-Verlag.

Trunnion Corrosion in Total Hip Arthroplasty—Basic Concepts

Kenneth L. Urish, MD, PhD[a,b,c,d,*],
Nicholas John Giori, MD, PhD[e,f,1], Jack E. Lemons, PhD[g],
William M. Mihalko, MD, PhD[h], Nadim Hallab, PhD[i]

KEYWORDS

- Corrosion • Trunnion • Adverse local tissue reaction • Total hip arthroplasty
- Head neck taper corrosion • Passive layer

KEY POINTS

- The passive layer serves a critical role in preventing corrosion on orthopedic implants.
- The femoral head-neck trunnion creates an optimal environment for corrosion to occur because of the limited fluid diffusion, acidic environment, and increased bending moment.

INTRODUCTION

Corrosion is electrochemical degradation of metallic materials and has been a central problem of orthopedics since metals were introduced as implantable biomaterials.[1] In this text, metals (elements), and alloys (combinations of elements) are called *metals*. As early as 1937, Venable and colleagues[2] were the first to report that Vitallium, a cobalt-chromium–based alloy, was superior to other metals (eg, aluminum, copper, iron, nickel, lead, gold, magnesium, silver, and iron-based alloys, such as stainless steels) in corrosion resistance and had adequate mechanical properties required for an implantable medical device. These early researchers observed the detrimental effects of corrosion on tissue and thus how corrosion-resistant alloys were paramount for orthopedic implants. This initial work set guidelines for the performance by which future metallic alloys were selected for use in hip arthroplasty and other types of implants. Since the introduction of modular hip implants in the 1960s, concerns regarding metal corrosion at these modular connections have been ever present.[3] These concerns were validated when galvanic, crevice, and fretting corrosion were observed and demonstrated in

Disclosure Statement: None.

Dr K. Urish is supported in part by the National Institute of Arthritis and Musculoskeletal and Skin Diseases (NIAMS K08AR071494), the National Center for Advancing Translational Sciences (NCATS KL2TR0001856), the Orthopaedic Research and Education Foundation, and the Musculoskeletal Transplant Foundation.

[a] Arthritis and Arthroplasty Design Group, The Bone and Joint Center, Magee Womens Hospital of the University of Pittsburgh Medical Center, 300 Halket Street, Suite 1601, Pittsburgh, PA 15213, USA; [b] Department of Orthopaedic Surgery, Clinical and Translational Science Institute, University of Pittsburgh, Pittsburgh, PA, USA; [c] Department of Bioengineering, Clinical and Translational Science Institute, University of Pittsburgh, Pittsburgh, PA, USA; [d] Department of Biomedical Engineering, Carnegie Mellon University, Pittsburgh, PA, USA; [e] VA Palo Alto Health Care System, Palo Alto, CA, USA; [f] Department of Orthopaedic Surgery, Stanford University, Stanford, CA, USA; [g] Department of Orthopaedic Surgery, University of Alabama at Birmingham, 1313 13th Street South, Birmingham, AL 35205-5327, USA; [h] Campbell Clinic, Department of Orthopaedic Surgery & Biomedical Engineering, University of Tennessee Health Science Center, 1211 Union Avenue, Suite 510, Memphis, TN 38104, USA; [i] Department of Orthopaedic Surgery, Rush University, 1653 West Congress Parkway, Chicago, IL 60612, USA

[1] Present address: 450 Broadway Street, Pavilion C, 4th Floor, Redwood City, CA 94063-6342.

* Corresponding author. 300 Halket Street, Suite 1601, Pittsburgh, PA 15213.

E-mail address: urishk2@upmc.edu

retrieved hip implants in the early 1990s.[4] Similarly, adverse tissues reactions, such as fibrous tissue masses, now termed, *adverse local tissue reactions (ALTRs)* or *pseudotumors*, were associated with head-neck trunnion corrosion as early as 1988.[5] The contribution of corrosion debris to the long-term performance of arthroplasty implants in general remains largely unknown.

Although metal-related tissue necrosis and implant revisions had been previously reported with historical metal-on-metal implants,[6] there was an increase in metal-on-metal bearing use in the early 2000s to mid-2000s, when surgeons tried to address problems associated with conventional polyethylene wear. Adverse metal-associated tissue reactions then reappeared as a source of poor implant performance in some arthroplasty designs.[7–10] Research in this area led to improved diagnostic tools, such as metal artifact reduction sequence MRI,[11] metal ion level tests,[12] and metal hypersensitivity tests.[13,14] Using these diagnostic tools, several investigations have noted that metal-associated tissue destruction, which was initially believed unique to metal-on-metal wear debris, could also be found in implants with metal-on-polyethylene bearings.[15–19] The degree to which these ALTRs in metal-on-metal hip replacements were due to metal wear debris from the articulation or from modular taper junction corrosion remains uncertain.[20,21]

Because modularity is part of almost all modern total hip arthroplasties, it is important that orthopedic surgeons understand how corrosion at these interfaces can determine implant outcome. This article reviews the basic concepts of corrosion thermodynamics on implant surfaces, the role of passive oxide layers in protecting the metal implant surfaces from corrosion, the various types and mechanisms of implant associated corrosion, and how these interact in the case of modular taper junctions to accelerate corrosion and decrease implant performance.

CORROSION BASIC SCIENCE

Corrosion is driven by thermodynamics for a material to go toward a lower chemical energy state and occurs when electrons flow from the anode (loss of electrons) to the cathode (gain of electrons). This is an exothermic process with minimal activation energy, which allows the reaction to occur spontaneously at either a fast or slow rate. When a bare metal surface without a protective metal-oxide film is directly exposed to air or an aqueous solution, the reaction is explosively exothermic. An excellent example of

this is titanium. Vacuum-processed titanium powder corrodes from a metallic state to an oxide at such a violent rate and with such a powerful release of energy that it has been used as solid rocket propellant. On the opposite end of this spectrum, ASTM titanium alloys have such a low rate of corrosion that they are an ideal material for many types of orthopedic implants. The difference in the rate of corrosion between vacuum processed titanium and ASTM titanium alloy is that ASTM titanium alloy rapidly forms a protective oxide film (also known as a passive layer) on its surface when it is exposed to oxygen. This process is known as *passivation*. This protective oxide film nearly stops corrosion on the surface of the metal, making a metal that can be used as a rocket propellant safe and stable for use as an implant.

Corrosion occurs in 3 basic steps (**Fig. 1**). First, metal from the surface dissolves into the aqueous environment and cations are removed (oxidation). Second, remaining electrons are attracted to a differential charge at another point on the surface. A current is generated as electrons are removed from the surface, driving the reaction (reduction). Finally, metal oxide or metal hydroxide form as byproducts. Metal oxides and insoluble metal hydroxides (rust) form an insulating layer on the metal surface. This precipitate forms a film that inhibits the kinetics of the reaction and insulates the metal from further corrosion.[22]

The passive chemically stable metal oxide layer is the key to preventing corrosion on orthopedic implants. Compared with metal hydroxide, the metal oxide is more stable, less soluble, and more insulating. Because the metal oxide film is nonconductive and an insulator, it prevents the flow of ions (current) from the solution's aqueous layer to the metal surface and thus limits the rate of corrosion. These films can only form with specific types of metal alloys. Stable passive metals include Ti, Cr, Ta, Nb, and Zr. Other metals, such as Al, Cu, In, and Tn, can form metal oxide layers, but these protective layers can quickly dissolve in the presence of chloride ions, a main constituent of physiologic solutions. Remaining elemental metal in alloys can corrode to form a metal hydroxide layer (ie, rust), which has a limited ability to prevent the movement of ions and limit corrosion.

Corrosion still occurs after passivation, but the passive film provides a large kinetic barrier slowing the speed of the reaction. The thermodynamics after passivation are changed because the activation energy is greatly increased with a passive barrier. This film forms almost instantly

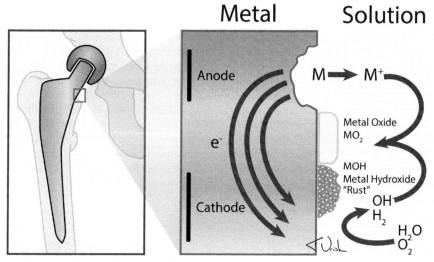

Fig. 1. Corrosion on a surface. In theory, maximum corrosion occurs if the complete metal surface was exposed on a surface. Corrosion occurs in 3 basic steps: (1) metal dissolves on the surface into the aqueous environment and cations are removed (oxidation); (2) remaining electrons are attracted to a differential charge at another point on the surface where electrons are removed from the metal driving the reaction (reduction); and (3) metal oxide or metal hydroxide form as byproducts of this reaction. Metal oxides and insoluble metal oxides (rust) form an insulating layer on the metal surface almost instantly that inhibit the kinetics of corrosion and insulate the metal from further corrosion. e^-, electrons; M, elemental metal; M^+, cationic metal ion; OH^-, hydroxide ion; H_2O, water; O_2, oxygen; H_2, hydrogen; MO_2, metal oxide; MOH, metal hydroxide.

on the surface of the metal. If the film remains homogenous and undisturbed, corrosion is inhibited as the uniform passive film shields the metal surface from the aqueous reaction (**Fig. 2**). Passive films prevent corrosion based on their properties, such as thickness and stability. This layer is not static and is in a constant steady state equilibrium. Its thickness is a balance between reactions that erode and build the film and a function of the voltage or electric field across the film and pH of the solution. A complete discussion of this is outside the scope of this discussion but reviewed elsewhere.[23]

TYPES OF CORROSION

The basic types of corrosion that can occur on an orthopedic implant include pitting, crevice,

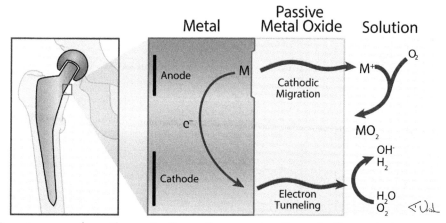

Fig. 2. Corrosion on a surface with a passive film—uniform corrosion. If a passive film remains homogenous and undisturbed, corrosion is inhibited as the uniform passive film shields the metal surface from the aqueous reaction. Metal oxide forms a stronger barrier to migration of the positive charged metal and electrons compared with the insoluble hydroxide (rust). The passive film thickness is a balance between reactions that erode and build the film. e^- electrons; M elemental metal; M^+ cationic metal ion; OH^- hydroxide ion; H_2O water; O_2 oxygen; H_2 hydrogen; MO_2 metal oxide; MOH metal hydroxide.

fretting, and mechanically assisted crevice corrosion (MACC). These different types of corrosion are all part of continuous spectrum based on a metal alloy's ability to avoid breakdown of the protective passivation layer. Pitting corrosion occurs from localized breakdown in the passive layer. Crevice corrosion is a form of pitting corrosion in a relatively harsher environment with limited mass transport. Fretting corrosion in a crevice is a form of MACC where crevice corrosion is facilitated by mechanical stress or mechanical motion. Fretting refers to low-amplitude mechanical wear of a surface; fretting corrosion refers to low amplitude wear of a metal surface where passivation layer removal takes place increasing metal degradation; and fretting corrosion in a crevice is more simply referred to as MACC.

Pitting corrosion is due to a localized relative dissolution of the passive film (Fig. 3), that is, where there is a small disruption on the passive film. This decreases the activation energy hurdle for corrosion, creating a more favorable environment for corrosion by speeding the kinetics in that area. Slight inconsistencies that develop and grow in the passive film lead to breakdown in small areas, which leads to the development of a focused anode, and localized galvanic corrosion.[24] For example, if 1 area of the passive film has a small amount of more permeable hydroxide than impermeable oxide, a defect can develop over this area of the passive surface (pitting). This creates a more permeable and less protective film. In aqueous solutions, halides (ie, Cl−) are readily available that can also help dissolve oxides and encourage less of an oxide barrier to form, allowing a larger flow of metal ions to escape from this small disrupted area. As a consequence, a differential cathode can develop over a large distant surface in response to the point anode. This creates a large difference in potential charge at 2 distant points. The current flow between these 2 charges is similar to the voltage difference across a battery and similar to galvanic corrosion.[24,25]

Crevice corrosion occurs, as the name implies, in a crevice where there is limited diffusion of ions in and out of the local environment, producing a harsher more corrosion-inducing environment (Fig. 4). Thus, as this crevice environment becomes more corrosive, compared with pitting corrosion, the activation energy is lower given the more favorable (eg, acidic) local conditions. Reaction kinetics are increased; however, the energy released (overall free energy) remains the same. The total hip arthroplasty trunnion is theoretically a closed environment that prevents ion diffusion (see Fig. 4). In practice, however, only a partial seal is established at a finite point on the neck-head taper connection, not across the entire taper surface. The trunnion occluded area becomes an obstacle preventing the diffusion of ions. Oxygen becomes depleted, limiting the ability of a passive layer to regenerate itself (repassivation). Hydrogen and chloride ion (hydrochloric acid) concentration increases. This creates a low acidic pH environment that accelerates corrosion by limiting repassivation. In this acidic crevice, the rate of corrosion is

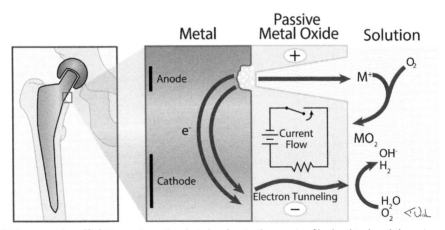

Fig. 3. Pitting corrosion. Slight inconsistencies that develop in the passive film lead to breakdown in small areas, development of a focused anode, and localized galvanic corrosion. A large flow of metal ions occurs at this focused anode. A differential cathode then develops over a large surface at a distant point. The current flow between these 2 charges is similar to the voltage difference across a battery or galvanic corrosion. e^- electrons; M elemental metal; M^+ cationic metal ion; OH^- hydroxide ion; H_2O water; O_2 oxygen; H_2 hydrogen; MO_2 metal oxide; MOH metal hydroxide.

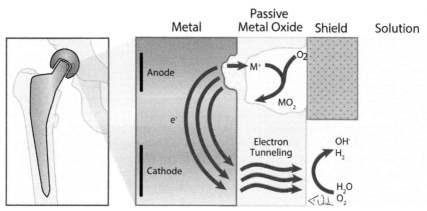

Fig. 4. Crevice corrosion. Pitting corrosion that occurs with limited diffusion of ions creates optimal conditions for corrosion. The total hip arthroplasty trunnion is a closed environment that prevents ion diffusion. A watertight seal is established at a finite point on the neck-head taper and prevents the diffusion of ions. Oxygen depletion and a low pH environment prevent repassivation. e^- electrons; M elemental metal; M^+ cationic metal ion; OH^- hydroxide ion; H_2O water; O_2 oxygen; H_2 hydrogen; MO_2 metal oxide; MOH metal hydroxide.

increased and the low concentration of oxygen limits metal oxide formation as a passive film. Simultaneously, there are increased chloride concentrations that further help increase the solubility of the passive film and decrease its stability. The resulting conditions in the trunnion crevice deteriorate to the points where the metal surface has a small inconsistent passive film that is not insulated from an aqueous solution. These are ideal conditions for corrosion.

As discussed previously, fretting corrosion in a crevice environment is considered MACC, that is combined crevice corrosion with additional mechanical disruption of the passive film with low-amplitude wear (**Fig. 5**). Tribocorrosion refers to the process of this combination of corrosion and wear combined.[26,27] Physical shearing forces remove the protective passive film that serves as

a barrier to corrosion for the metal surface. At the taper interface, small oscillations between the taper surfaces can act to remove passive film and thus cause significant fretting corrosion or MACC. Increased head sizes, smaller and more flexible trunnions, and smaller trunnion contact areas all act to increase the local shear forces across the taper junction and thus increase the potential for MACC. In the context of trunnion corrosion, both fretting corrosion and MACC are terms generally used interchangeably despite that fretting corrosion need not take place in a crevice environment.

TRUNNION CORROSION

Trunnion design parameters play a critical role that contribute to passive film instability. A Morse

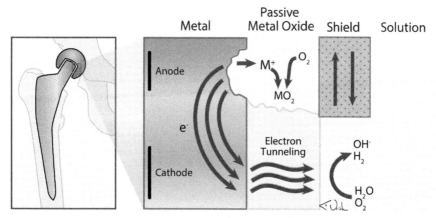

Fig. 5. Fretting corrosion or MACC. A physical shearing force across the trunnion removes the protective passive film. This creates a larger surface for crevice corrosion to occur. e^- electrons; M elemental metal; M^+ cationic metal ion; OH^- hydroxide ion; H_2O water; O_2 oxygen; H_2 hydrogen; MO_2 metal oxide; MOH metal hydroxide.

taper is defined by the angle that the taper surfaces make relative to the longitudinal axis of the component.[28] These taper design parameters (length, slope, and angle) and the elastic modulus of the metal affect the overall structural rigidity. For example, for 2 theoretic trunnions of identical metal alloy, the trunnion with the shorter mating surface and narrow diameter is the more flexible. Theoretically, this produces more fretting movement and consequent MACC. This has led to multiple groups suggesting that changes in trunnion geometry with smaller diameters and shorter taper length are important factors in predicting trunnion corrosion.[29–33] At what point these theoretic design parameters reach a threshold to make an implant more susceptible to corrosion in the highly complex in vivo environment remains unclear.

The magnitude of mechanical stress across the trunnion also may affect passive film stability. Larger femoral head diameters and longer neck length femoral heads may cause greater material deformation at the taper junction and thus more relative motion between the 2 mating surfaces. These clinical generalizations are evidence based on a series of retrieval studies that suggest larger head sizes are associated with increased incidence of ALTR.[34–37] Other models have suggested head-neck offset would increase micromotion.[38] Taper geometry and contact length also are known to play key roles in controlling trunnion corrosion. In vivo, the femoral head does not make contact with the entire mating surface of the femoral stem across the surface of the trunnion. Thus, the smaller the contact area, the more stress placed across the trunnion surface. Furthermore, there is variation in surface topology across different tapers,[39] with some tapers having grooved surfaces whereas others having smoother surfaces. It is generally accepted that increased mechanical stress and movement across the trunnion interface due to various prosthetic design features result in accelerated corrosion and an increase of ALTR.[40,41]

The stability of the passive film is essential to limit corrosion from the optimized highly corrosive environment. The oxide film that forms on the passive layer prevents the dissolution of the metal ions and can regenerate itself if disrupted. Tribocorrosion has the synergistic ability to accelerate corrosion from the mechanical wear across the passive film. Trunnion design parameters, such as taper length, diameter, contact area, and mechanical stress, across the trunnion interface may accelerate corrosion and lead to ALTR but the interplay of these factors, including surgical technique, remains to be determined.

Arthroplasty surgeons should be aware of these issues and how to limit the possibility of corrosion. Modularity should be minimized where possible, especially if minimal or no advantages to wear or stability result. Femoral head material can have an affect on the amount of corrosion that may occur at the taper, and, if possible and cost effective, ceramic heads should be considered.[42] During femoral head and trunnion assembly, care should be taken to make certain the trunnion is dry and void of any debris before assembly. Although many manufacturers do not offer optimal assembly technique guides,[43] it has been determined that an axially directed force of over 2.5 kN should be used to optimize the modular connection between the head and trunnion of the stem.[44] When dealing with a revision scenario for a corroded trunnion, it has been shown that cleaning the trunnion and placing a new femoral head (cobalt-chromium or ceramic) has no difference in stability of the head trunnion junction compared to pristine new tapers.[45] In a revision scenario for ALTR, ceramic heads should be highly considered. Surgeons should also make certain after they assemble the femoral head trunnion connection or after they implant total knee arthroplasty components that the electrocautery should not be placed on or near the cobalt-chromium–bearing surfaces. The plasma discharge can disrupt the oxide layer of the bearing and cause pits on the surface.[46,47] These simple pearls can help surgeons optimize and reduce the risk of corrosion related factors to obtain the best environment and scenario for a good long-term outcome.

REFERENCES

1. Ferguson AB Jr, Laing PG, Hodge ES. The ionization of metal implants in living tissues. J Bone Joint Surg Am 1960;42-A:77.
2. Venable CS, Stuck WG, Beach A. The effects on bone of the presence of metals; based upon electrolysis: an experimental study. Ann Surg 1937; 105(6):917.
3. Collier JP, Mayor MB, Jensen RE, et al. Mechanisms of failure of modular prostheses. Clin Orthop Relat Res 1992;(285):129.
4. Gilbert JL, Buckley CA, Jacobs JJ. In vivo corrosion of modular hip prosthesis components in mixed and similar metal combinations. The effect of crevice, stress, motion, and alloy coupling. J Biomed Mater Res 1993;27(12):1533.
5. Svensson O, Mathiesen EB, Reinholt FP, et al. Formation of a fulminant soft-tissue pseudotumor

after uncemented hip arthroplasty. A case report. J Bone Joint Surg Am 1988;70(8):1238.

6. Evans EM, Freeman MA, Miller AJ, et al. Metal sensitivity as a cause of bone necrosis and loosening of the prosthesis in total joint replacement. J Bone Joint Surg Br 1974;56-B(4):626.

7. Clayton RA, Beggs I, Salter DM, et al. Inflammatory pseudotumor associated with femoral nerve palsy following metal-on-metal resurfacing of the hip. A case report. J Bone Joint Surg Am 2008; 90(9):1988.

8. Counsell A, Heasley R, Arumilli B, et al. A groin mass caused by metal particle debris after hip resurfacing. Acta Orthop Belg 2008;74(6):870.

9. Mahendra G, Pandit H, Kliskey K, et al. Necrotic and inflammatory changes in metal-on-metal resurfacing hip arthroplasties. Acta Orthop 2009;80(6):653.

10. Campbell P, Ebramzadeh E, Nelson S, et al. Histological features of pseudotumor-like tissues from metal-on-metal hips. Clin Orthop Relat Res 2010; 468(9):2321.

11. Gottlob I, Stangler-Zuschrott E. Effect of levodopa on contrast sensitivity and scotomas in human amblyopia. Invest Ophthalmol Vis Sci 1990;31(4):776.

12. Campbell PA, Kung MS, Hsu AR, et al. Do retrieval analysis and blood metal measurements contribute to our understanding of adverse local tissue reactions? Clin Orthop Relat Res 2014;472(12):3718.

13. Bravo D, Wagner ER, Larson DR, et al. No increased risk of knee arthroplasty failure in patients with positive skin patch testing for metal hypersensitivity: a matched cohort study. J Arthroplasty 2016;31(8): 1717.

14. Thomas P, von der Helm C, Schopf C, et al. Patients with intolerance reactions to total knee replacement: combined assessment of allergy diagnostics, periprosthetic histology, and peri-implant cytokine expression pattern. Biomed Res Int 2015;2015: 910156.

15. Fricka KB, Ho H, Peace WJ, et al. Metal-on-metal local tissue reaction is associated with corrosion of the head taper junction. J Arthroplasty 2012; 27(8 Suppl):26.

16. Plummer DR, Berger RA, Paprosky WG, et al. Diagnosis and management of adverse local tissue reactions secondary to corrosion at the head-neck junction in patients with metal on polyethylene bearings. J Arthroplasty 2016;31(1):264.

17. McGrory BJ, MacKenzie J, Babikian G. A high prevalence of corrosion at the head-neck taper with contemporary zimmer non-cemented femoral hip components. J Arthroplasty 2015; 30(7):1265.

18. Fehring TK, Fehring K, Odum SM. Metal artifact reduction sequence MRI abnormalities occur in metal-on-polyethylene hips. Clin Orthop Relat Res 2015;473(2):574.

19. Urish KL, Hamlin BR, Plakseychuk AY, et al. Trunnion failure of the recalled low friction ion treatment cobalt chromium alloy femoral head. J Arthroplasty 2017;32(9):2857.

20. Cook RB, Bolland BJ, Wharton JA, et al. Pseudotumour formation due to tribocorrosion at the taper interface of large diameter metal on polymer modular total hip replacements. J Arthroplasty 2013;28(8):1430.

21. Jacobs JJ, Cooper HJ, Urban RM, et al. What do we know about taper corrosion in total hip arthroplasty? J Arthroplasty 2014;29(4):668.

22. Jacobs JJ, Gilbert JL, Urban RM. Corrosion of metal orthopaedic implants. J Bone Joint Surg Am 1998;80(2):268.

23. Macdonald DD. The history of the point defect model for the passive state: a brief review of film growth aspects. Electrochim Acta 2011;56(4):1761.

24. Szklarska-Smialowska Z, National Association of Corrosion Engineers. Pitting corrosion of metals. Houston (TX): National Association of Corrosion Engineers; 1986.

25. Hodgson AW, Mischler S, Von Rechenberg B, et al. An analysis of the in vivo deterioration of Co-Cr-Mo implants through wear and corrosion. Proc Inst Mech Eng H 2007;221(3):291.

26. Munoz AI, Mischler S. Interactive effects of albumin and phosphate ions on the corrosion of CoCrMo implant alloy. J Electrochem Soc 2007;154(10):C562.

27. Wimmer MA, Fischer A, Buscher R, et al. Wear mechanisms in metal-on-metal bearings: the importance of tribochemical reaction layers. J Orthop Res 2010;28(4):436.

28. Lucas LC, Buchanan RA, Lemons JE. Investigations on the galvanic corrosion of multialloy total hip prostheses. J Biomed Mater Res 1981;15(5):731.

29. Brown SA, Flemming CA, Kawalec JS, et al. Fretting corrosion accelerates crevice corrosion of modular hip tapers. J Appl Biomater 1995;6(1):19.

30. Goldberg JR, Gilbert JL, Jacobs JJ, et al. A multicenter retrieval study of the taper interfaces of modular hip prostheses. Clin Orthop Relat Res 2002;(401):149.

31. Grupp TM, Weik T, Bloemer W, et al. Modular titanium alloy neck adapter failures in hip replacement— failure mode analysis and influence of implant material. BMC Musculoskelet Disord 2010;11:3.

32. Brock TM, Sidaginamale R, Rushton S, et al. Shorter, rough trunnion surfaces are associated with higher taper wear rates than longer, smooth trunnion surfaces in a contemporary large head metal-on-metal total hip arthroplasty system. J Orthop Res 2015;33(12):1868.

33. Nassif NA, Nawabi DH, Stoner K, et al. Taper design affects failure of large-head metal-on-metal total hip replacements. Clin Orthop Relat Res 2014; 472(2):564.

34. Bishop N, Witt F, Pourzal R, et al. Wear patterns of taper connections in retrieved large diameter metal-on-metal bearings. J Orthop Res 2013;31(7):1116.

35. Bolland BJ, Culliford DJ, Langton DJ, et al. High failure rates with a large-diameter hybrid metal-on-metal total hip replacement: clinical, radiological and retrieval analysis. J Bone Joint Surg Br 2011;93(5):608.

36. Langton D, Ahmed I, Avery P, et al. Investigation of taper failure in a contemporary metal-on-metal hip arthroplasty system through examination of unused and explanted prostheses. J Bone Joint Surg Am 2017;99(5):427.

37. Dyrkacz RM, Brandt JM, Ojo OA, et al. The influence of head size on corrosion and fretting behaviour at the head-neck interface of artificial hip joints. J Arthroplasty 2013;28(6):1036.

38. Donaldson FE, Coburn JC, Siegel KL. Total hip arthroplasty head-neck contact mechanics: a stochastic investigation of key parameters. J Biomech 2014;47(7):1634.

39. Munir S, Walter WL, Walsh WR. Variations in the trunnion surface topography between different commercially available hip replacement stems. J Orthop Res 2015;33(1):98.

40. Lavernia CJ, Iacobelli DA, Villa JM, et al. Trunnion-head stresses in THA: are big heads trouble? J Arthroplasty 2015;30(6):1085.

41. Weiser MC, Lavernia CJ. Trunnionosis in total hip arthroplasty. J Bone Joint Surg Am 2017;99(17):1489.

42. Wyles CC, McArthur BA, Wagner ER, et al. Ceramic femoral heads for all patients? An argument for cost containment in hip surgery. Am J Orthop (Belle Mead NJ) 2016;45(6):E362.

43. McGrory BJ, Ng E. No consensus for femoral head impaction technique in surgeon education materials from orthopedic implant manufacturers. J Arthroplasty 2018;33(6):1749–51.e1.

44. Ramoutar DN, Crosnier EA, Shivji F, et al. Assessment of head displacement and disassembly force with increasing assembly load at the head/trunnion junction of a total hip arthroplasty prosthesis. J Arthroplasty 2017;32(5):1675.

45. Derasari A, Gold JE, Ismaily S, et al. Will new metal heads restore mechanical integrity of corroded trunnions? J Arthroplasty 2017;32(4):1356.

46. Yuan N, Park SH, Luck JV Jr, et al. Revisiting the concept of inflammatory cell-induced corrosion. J Biomed Mater Res B Appl Biomater 2018;106(3):1148–55.

47. Kubacki GW, Sivan S, Gilbert JL. Electrosurgery induced damage to Ti-6Al-4V and CoCrMo alloy surfaces in orthopedic implants in vivo and in vitro. J Arthroplasty 2017;32(11):3533.

Trauma

Suprapatellar Tibial Nailing

Gennadiy A. Busel, MD, Hassan Mir, MD, MBA*

KEYWORDS

- Suprapatellar • Semiextended • Tibia fracture • Intramedullary nail

---

KEY POINTS

- Suprapatellar nailing portal eliminates the need for hyperflexion during tibial nailing and manipulation of the limb during fluoroscopy.
- Leg positioning allows for improved trajectory for guide wire placement.
- Suprapatellar tibial nailing decreased the rates of malreduction in proximal and distal third tibia shaft fractures.
- Specific instrumentation is required for suprapatellar nailing. Surgeons must be aware of the differences in instrumentation between suprapatellar and infrapatellar nailing techniques.

HISTORY

The treatment of tibia shaft fractures has progressed from casting and functional bracing to intramedullary fixation, as developed by Küntscher in 1940s.[1] The first intramedullary devices were reliant on diaphyseal fit because interlocking screws did not exist, thus limiting rotational control. This design limitation restricted the application of these implants to length-stable diaphyseal fractures. With the advent of interlocking screws, control of rotation and shortening became possible expanding the use of the intramedullary nail to include a variety of unstable fractures of the tibia. Today, intramedullary nailing of the tibia is the preferred treatment method, performed across the United States and the globe.

Although nailing of the tibia has become the gold standard, problems were encountered with fixation of proximal metaphyseal fractures.[2] The importance of the starting point and the guide wire trajectory has been researched thoroughly in literature.[3,4] Reaching that ideal starting point, however, has been problematic in the past with the use of either a patellar tendon-splitting or tendon-sparing approach. This necessitated hyperflexion of the knee over a triangle to clear the patella and obtain adequate guide wire trajectory. The required hyperflexion gave rise to 2 unintended problems. First, obtaining fluoroscopic assessment of the starting point in the coronal plane required significant tilting of the C-arm, which is often limited by the bottom of the operating table. Second, and more important, the pull of the quadriceps as well as posteriorly directed nail caused flexion in the proximal segment, resulting in a well-described, procurvatum deformity (**Fig. 1**).[2]

Numerous techniques have been developed to combat these problems, including provisional plating and use of blocking screws.[5,6] In 1996 Tornetta and Collins[7] described a semiextended position for tibial nailing as a potential solution to the problem. The article highlighted nailing of the tibia with the knee at approximately 15° to 20° of flexion through a medial parapatellar arthrotomy. This allowed lateral mobilization of the patella, permitting easy access to the appropriate starting point, all the while maintaining the extensor mechanism relaxed. Although successful results have been demonstrated with this approach, concerns for extensive dissection and a need for an arthrotomy led to modifications of this technique. Kubiak and colleagues[8] described an extra-articular modification, whereas other investigators expanded on the idea of semiextended nailing by proposing a

---

Disclosure Statement: The authors have nothing to disclose.
Department of Orthopaedic Surgery, Florida Orthopaedic Institute, 5 Tampa General Circle, Suite 710, Tampa, FL 33606, USA
* Corresponding author.
E-mail address: hmir@floridaortho.com

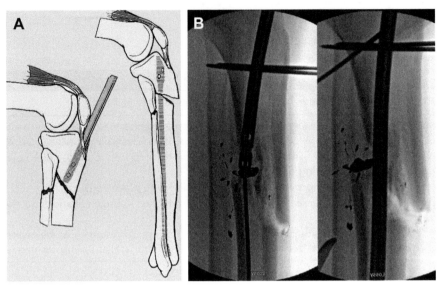

Fig. 1. (A) Image illustrates initial aim of the nail posteriorly and resulting procurvatum deformity. (B) Clinical image of procurvatum deformity after tibial nailing.

suprapatellar entry portal (Dean Cole personal communications[9]). Although the leap from a semiextended, parapatellar approach to the suprapatellar portal may now seem intuitive, limitation in availability of the appropriate instrumentation caused a significant delay in its implementation.

BENEFIT OF THE TECHNIQUE

There are numerous benefits to the semiextended suprapatellar tibial nailing. The 2 advantages discussed previously are extensor mechanism relaxation and improved guide wire trajectory, as too posterior a nail trajectory leads to procurvatum. As demonstrated by Eastman and colleagues,[10] a retropatellar technique allowed for a more favorable sagittal plane insertion angle compared with infrapatellar approach (Fig. 2). Furthermore, semiextended positioning allows for ease of radiographs in both anteroposterior (AP) and lateral views without manipulation of the extremity. The ability to maintain the leg in a static position throughout the entire procedure led to improvement with nailing of the distal metaphyseal tibia fractures as well. Avilucea and colleagues[11] found that the rate of malalignment of distal one-third tibia fractures decreased from 26.1% to 3.8% compared with infrapatellar technique. The group highlighted the ease of maintaining the reduction, once achieved, during reaming and nail passage as the major factor for improved outcome.

Finally, a study evaluating the amount of anterior cortical bone removal and potential injury to the intermeniscal ligament at the tibial entry zone found that suprapatellar entry portal led to a decreased incidence of damage to intraarticular structures.[12]

TECHNIQUE/INSTRUMENTATION

The patient is positioned supine on a radiolucent table. Some investigators use this time to examine the patellar laxity of the injured extremity. Although not always accurate, this can provide information for a possible need for extended release (discussed later). Alternatively, contralateral uninjured patellar mobility may be used preoperatively for the same reason. A hip bump under the involved extremity is used to assist with internal rotation of the leg to allow the patella to face directly anterior. The leg is placed on a leg ramp to allow for a lateral radiograph without interference from the contralateral limb. The ramp is secured to the bed to prevent displacement. Tourniquet, if used, is placed in a nonsterile fashion, making sure the drape is placed in such a way as to keep the distal half of the thigh exposed. It is the preferred technique of the authors to shave the area proximal to the patella, if applicable. After draping, a knee bolster is used to obtain approximately 15° of knee flexion to allow access to the proximal tibia for a correct starting point (Fig. 3).

The superior pole of the patella is identified. An approximately 2-cm skin incision is marked in the midline starting a fingerbreadth above the patella and extending proximal (Fig. 4).

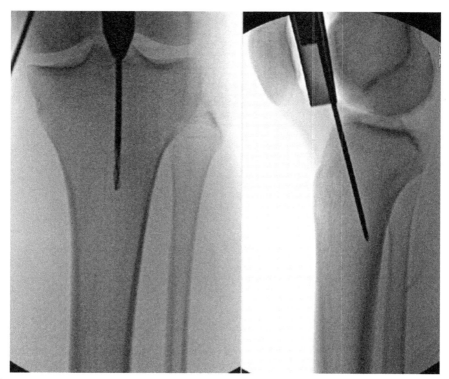

Fig. 2. Starting trajectory using a suprapatellar entry portal on AP and lateral radiographs.

Sharp dissection is carried down to the quadriceps muscle, which is easily identified. A full-thickness incision is made in the midsubstance of the quadriceps tendon, stopping 5 mm short of the superior pole of the patella, thus entering the knee joint. Finger palpation is used to assess the tightness of the patellofemoral joint for ease of trocar insertion. A retractor can be used to elevate the patella, if needed. Should the patellofemoral space be deemed too tight for safe trocar insertion, mobility of the patella can be assessed to see which direction, medial or lateral, it can be more easily subluxated. A medial or lateral patellar retinacular release is performed, allowing the respective subluxation/mobilization of the patella. A cuff of tissue should be left intact for later repair of the extensor mechanism during closure. A trocar is inserted in a retropatellar fashion, ensuring the cannula is down to the tibia, protecting the femoral condyles and patellar cartilage from damage during reaming. The cannula can be either pinned in place to the femur, if the system allows it, to prevent pistoning during reaming and thus damaging the articular cartilage with the edge of the cannula, or routinely checked that it is pushed down all the way throughout the procedure. Surgeons should be familiar with the instrumentation because certain companies have 2 trocars of different diameters. The larger trocar allows for reaming and nail insertion to be done without the removal of the trocar (based on size of the nail); however, the smaller trocar does not allow for the passage

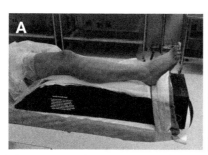
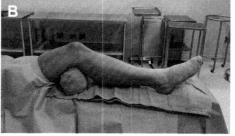

Fig. 3. (A) Preparation and (B) Positioning of the involved extremity.

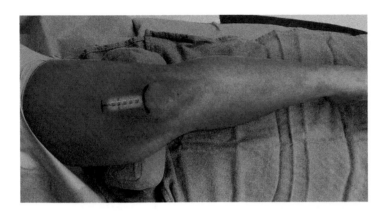

Fig. 4. Landmarks and planned incision. Dotted line represents incision; solid line is proximal extent if needed.

of the nail and requires removal. If the larger trocar does not have adequate room to be inserted, the smaller one may be used, thus foregoing the patellar retinacular release whenever possible.

Once the cannula is confirmed to be down to the tibia, a guide wire is inserted through the central opening. As is typical for intramedullary nailing of the tibia, fluoroscopy should be used to assess for appropriate starting position. Numerous investigators have described appropriate starting point.[3,4,13] It should be medial to the lateral tibial spine, as viewed on the AP radiograph, and just anterior to the articular surface, as seen on the lateral image. The surgeon should be careful to obtain adequate AP and lateral radiographs because the starting point may appear falsely accurate if nonstandard fluoroscopy is viewed.[14] Bible and colleagues[15] compared tibia-based referencing for proximal tibia radiographs and showed that a fibular head bisection and twin peaks AP images are safe for a starting point. In a fibular head bisection image, the fibular head should be seen as divided in 2 by the lateral tibial plateau, whereas the twin peaks AP image shows the sharpest profile of the tibial spines. As for the lateral, either femoral condyle overlap or flat plateau can be used safely. In either of the lateral views, femoral condyles or tibial plateaus should be aligned to show a single silhouette, respectively. Investigators have noted that although no difference in intra-articular damage existed between the 2, twin peaks AP radiograph was externally rotated by $2.7° \pm 2.1°$ compared with fibular head bisector image.[15]

As shown previously, too medial a starting point can create valgus, in the proximal one-third tibia fractures, whereas too lateral a start can cause varus. Similarly, too posterior a trajectory can kick the proximal segment into procurvatum. This highlights the importance of an appropriate starting point and that the surgeons should not accept anything short of a perfect guide wire placement. If the initial guide wire placement is suboptimal, it can be left in and used as a reference with assistance of a honeycomb inner cannula. Furthermore, it is not uncommon to be too steep with the entry guide wire, especially in the proximal tibia fractures. In this situation, an opening reamer can be used to open only a first few centimeters of the canal and an intramedullary reduction tool could be used to correct the trajectory (**Fig. 5**). Introduction of the reduction tool not only is useful in correction of the trajectory but also in aiding reduction of the fracture. Alternatively, the cannula may be hindering the ideal starting point by forcing a bad pin trajectory. In this situation, the authors recommend utilizing the guide wire–first technique, where the surgeon performs the approach and places the guide pin without the cannula in the ideal location. Subsequently, the cannula is slid over the pin for the protection of the patellofemoral joint (**Fig. 6**). As with most nailing of the long bones, the fracture must be reduced prior to canal reaming and nail insertion unless the fracture is isthmic and the nail is used for reduction.

Finally, suprapatellar entry portal technique requires awareness of another instrument variation: longer reamers or reamer extensions. The lengths of the flexible reamers vary; however, if the goal is to ream all the way to the distal physis, a reamer extension or longer reamer may be required if the tibia measures more than 340 mm. The depth of the reamer can easily be checked on the fluoroscopic imaging during the first pass and a decision made regarding the need for the extension. Conversely, some companies have longer reamers designed specifically for suprapatellar nailing that thus should

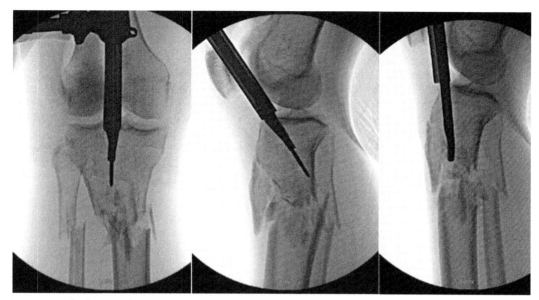

Fig. 5. Use of a finger reduction tool to correct the trajectory of the starting guide wire. Opening the canal minimally with the reamer (left and middle panel) with the subsequent use of the finger reduction tool to correct the trajectory of the starting guidewire (right panel).

be available in the operating room prior to the start of the case.

Irrigation of the joint and layered closure is done in a similar fashion as with other surgical interventions. Heavy absorbable suture is used for closure of the quadriceps tendon. Postoperative protocol does not vary between suprapatellar and infrapatellar entry portals and is instead based on surgeon preference and fracture pattern.

POTENTIAL RISKS

The main concern arising from the use of the suprapatellar nailing technique is the potential damage to the patellofemoral joint. Cadaveric model comparison looking at patellofemoral contact pressures with suprapatellar versus infrapatellar nailing techniques did find a difference between the 2.[16] The mean pressure of 2.13 MPa (range of 1.10–2.86 MPa), however, was significantly lower than that required to cause cartilage damage with a single impact (>25 MPa) or from sustained load (4.5 MPa). Similarly, clinical studies failed to find any clinical or radiographic complications associated with suprapatellar nailing. Sanders and colleagues[17] evaluated patients undergoing intramedullary nailing of the tibia in the semiextended approach through the suprapatellar portal

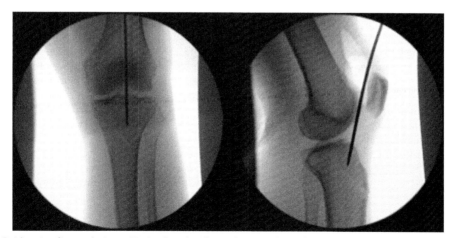

Fig. 6. Guide wire–first technique. Pin is placed without the cannula and the cannula is placed over the pin after ideal starting point is reached.

at minimum of 1-year follow-up. The investigators not only provided functional outcome scores but also obtained MRI scans as well as arthroscopic images in a (subgroup of study patients) of prenail and postnail insertions. Musculoskeletal radiologists reviewed MRIs whereas arthroscopic images were evaluated by an orthopedic sports medicine surgeons to eliminate bias. This study revealed no patellofemoral joint damage or clinical complications with the use of suprapatellar entry portal. Other investigators reproducing the same results have corroborated these findings further.[18] Sebest and colleagues[18] looked at pain and functional scores after suprapatellar nailing and evaluated patients with arthroscopy as well. The investigators reached the same conclusion as Sanders and colleagues,[17] stating that suprapatellar approach was not associated with either anterior knee pain or functional limitations. Both studies demonstrated absence of anterior knee pain often found with tibial nailing during standard, infrapatellar insertion technique. Five-year follow-up studies are in progress to provide longer-term outcomes of suprapatellar nailing.

Finally, just as a retrograde femur nailing is safe in open fractures and through a traumatic arthrotomy,[9] suprapatellar nailing also can be used in these situations.

An infrapatellar starting point still may serve a role in certain situations. Severe patellofemoral arthritis may be an indication to use infrapatellar portal because extensive soft tissue release with mobilization of patella almost certainly would be required.

SUMMARY

The suprapatellar nailing technique is an important adjunct in the armamentarium of an orthopedic surgeon. Although a variety of new instrumentations are required for insertion of the suprapatellar nail, most companies now carry these instruments. Easier positioning, maintenance of reduction, ease of intraoperative fluoroscopy, more anatomic starting trajectory, decreased malreduction rates, and possible decrease in anterior knee pain are all benefits of suprapatellar nailing, thus making mastery of this technique essential for an orthopedic surgeon.

REFERENCES

1. Bohler L. Medullary nailing of Kuntscher. 1st edition. Baltimore (MD): Williams and Wilkins; 1948.
2. Freedman EL, Johnson EE. Radiographic analysis of tibial fracture malalignment following intramedullary nailing. Clin Orthop Relat Res 1995;315:25–33.
3. Tornetta P 3rd, Riina J, Geller J, et al. Intra-articular anatomic risks of tibial nailing. J Orthop Trauma 1999;13:247–51.
4. Samuelson MA, McPherson EJ, Norris L. Anatomic assessment of the proper insertion site for a tibial intramedullary nail. J Orthop Trauma 2002;16:23–5.
5. Krettek C, Miclau T, Schandelmaier P, et al. The mechanical effect of blocking screws ("Poller screws") in stabilizing tibia fractures with short proximal or distal fragments after insertion of small-diameter intramedullary nails. J Orthop Trauma 1999;13:550–3.
6. Ricci WM, O'Boyle M, Borrelli J, et al. Fractures of the proximal third of the tibial shaft treated with intramedullary nails and blocking screws. J Orthop Trauma 2001;15:264–70.
7. Tornetta P, Collins E. Semiextended position of intramedullary nailing of the proximal tibia. Clin Orthop Relat Res 1996;(328):185–9.
8. Kubiak E, Widmer B, Horwitz D. Extra-articular technique for semiextended tibial nailing. J Orthop Trauma 2010;24:704–8.
9. O'Toole R, Riche K, Cannada L, et al. Analysis of postoperative knee sepsis after retrograde nail insertion of open femoral shaft fractures. J Orthop Trauma 2010;24(11):677–82.
10. Eastman J, Tseng S, Lo E, et al. Retropatellar technique for intramedullary nailing of proximal tibia fractures: a cadaveric assessment. J Orthop Trauma 2010;24:672–6.
11. Avilucea F, Triantafillou K, Whiting P, et al. Suprapatellar intramedullary nail technique lowers rate of malalignment of distal tibia fractures. J Orthop Trauma 2016;30:557–60.
12. Bible J, Choxie A, Dhulipala S, et al. Quantification of anterior cortical bone removal and intermeniscal ligament damage at the tibial nail entry zone using parapatellar and retropatellar approaches. J Orthop Trauma 2013;27:437–41.
13. McConnell T, Tornetta P, Tilzey J, et al. Tibial portal placement: the radiographic correlate of the anatomic safe zone. J Orthop Trauma 2001;15(3):2007–9.
14. Walker R, Zdero R, McKee M, et al. Ideal tibial intramedullary nail insertion point varies with tibial rotation. J Orthop Trauma 2011;25:726–30.
15. Bible J, Choxi A, Dhulipala S, et al. Tibia-based referencing for standard proximal tibial radiographs during intramedullary nailing. Am J Orthop (Belle Mead NJ) 2013;42(11):E95–8.
16. Gelbke MK, Coombs D, Powell S, et al. Suprapatellar versus infra-patellar intramedullary nail insertion of the tibia: a cadaveric model for comparison of

patellofemoral contact pressures and forces. J Orthop Trauma 2010;24:665–71.

17. Sanders R, DiPasquale T, Jordan C, et al. Semi-extended intramedullary nailing of the tibia using a suprapatellar approach: radiographic results and clinical outcomes at a minimum of 12 months follow-up. J Orthop Trauma 2014;28: S29–39.

18. Serbest S, TiftiKci U, Coban M, et al. Knee pain and functional scores after intramedullary nailing of tibial shaft fractures using a suprapatellar approach. J Orthop Trauma 2019;33(1):37–41.

The Reamer-Irrigator-Aspirator in Nonunion Surgery

Randall Drew Madison, MD*, Peter J. Nowotarski, MD

KEYWORDS

• Reamer-Irrigator-Aspirator • Nonunion • Autograft • Masquelet • Induced membrane

KEY POINTS

• Reamer-irrigator-aspirator (RIA) autograft possesses osteogenic, osteoinductive, and osteoconductive properties comparable to that of iliac crest bone graft.
• RIA autograft consistently and efficiently provides large volumes of autograft with less donor site morbidity than iliac crest bone graft.
• Use of RIA autograft has been demonstrated to produce similar successful union rates for segmental bone defects when compared with iliac crest bone graft.

INTRODUCTION

Although the first reports of intramedullary nailing date back to sixteenth century Mexico, its viability was not well established until the 1940s. Gerhard Küntscher, considered by many to be the godfather of contemporary intramedullary nailing, popularized the technique with his work during World War II. By extension, Küntscher's later introduction of motorized flexible reamers to allow larger-diameter nails led to concerns over increased intramedullary canal pressures and the morbidities associated with fat embolism.[1] Although Küntscher recognized the problem and offered technical guidelines to minimize canal pressure in the 1940s, it was not until 1970 and the publication by Danckwardt-Lilliestrom and colleagues[2] that the benefits of canal pressure reduction during reaming were detailed. However, it was not until the introduction of the "reamer-irrigator-aspirator" (RIA) system (Synthes, West Chester, PA) in 2001 that a commercial product was available for clinical use.

The RIA was designed to reduce the intramedullary canal pressure by providing continuous suction throughout the reaming process to reduce embolic load. The fenestrated reamer head provides a means by which to deliver irrigation to the cutting edge of the reamer with the intent of reducing temperature and the potential for thermal necrosis. The intramedullary contents, including irrigation fluid, bony fragments, and marrow, are evacuated under suction aspiration through the device in an attempt to reduce intramedullary canal pressures.[3]

Perhaps even more clinically useful than the RIA system's ability to reduce canal pressure, temperature, and embolic load, has been the expansion of its application in recent years to include autologous bone graft harvest. By simply adding a closed, inline filter and collection device, large volumes of autogenous endosteal intramedullary reaming graft material can be easily obtained. Before the RIA's introduction, early attempts at obtaining autograft via intramedullary reaming were somewhat successful. However, with no device to efficiently collect

Disclosure Statement: Dr R.D. Madison has nothing to disclose. Dr P.J. Nowotarski is a paid consultant for Depuy-Synthes for the development of the Femoral Reconstruction Nail System.
Division of Orthopaedic Trauma Surgery, University of Tennessee College of Medicine at Chattanooga/Erlanger Health System, 979 East 3rd Street, Suite C-225, Chattanooga, TN 37403, USA
* Corresponding author.
E-mail address: Drew.Madison.DM@gmail.com

reaming debris, intramedullary graft harvest proved technically demanding and yielded relatively low volumes of graft material.[4] In part, these struggles served to secure the role of cancellous iliac crest bone graft (ICBG) as the gold standard for autograft harvest. However, in the years since its introduction, RIA has become a safe, reliable, and efficient source of autograft.[5]

BIOLOGY OF REAMER-IRRIGATOR-ASPIRATOR AUTOGRAFT

Autogenous bone grafting has long been the preferred method in the treatment of nonunions and segmental defects. It offers osteogenic, osteoinductive, and osteoconductive properties while maintaining complete histocompatibility with no risk of disease transmission. In the past, both anterior and posterior ICBG have been heavily used and remain the gold standard against which all other grafts are measured; however, donor site morbidity and limited graft volume continue to be noteworthy shortcomings of ICBG.[6,7]

Several studies have advocated for the intramedullary canal as a viable source of autograft. These studies confirmed the presence of viable osteoblasts, osteocytes, and growth factors known to participate in osteogenesis and fracture healing.[8,9] Composed of 2 separate microenvironments known as the vascular and osteoblastic "niches," the intramedullary canal houses both hematopoietic stem cells and mesenchymal stem cells (MSCs). It has been suggested that the intramedullary canal and the endothelial beds of its vascular niche can offer a greater number of MSCs than can ICBG.[10] Sagi and colleagues[11] assessed both qualitative and quantitative differences by directly comparing bone graft obtained from the medullary canal and iliac crest of the same patient. They found that RIA samples contained more MSCs and exhibited significantly higher levels of expression of bone morphogenic proteins (BMPs) and vascular endothelial growth factor (VEGF) receptors. These results would suggest that RIA offers superior osteogenic and osteoinductive properties and equivalent osteoconductive properties when compared with ICBG.

MANAGING NONUNIONS AND SEGMENTAL DEFECTS WITH THE REAMER-IRRIGATOR-ASPIRATOR AUTOGRAFT

Critical evaluation of the history, physical examination, radiographs, and laboratory studies are paramount in the successful treatment of nonunions. Before devising a treatment strategy, the pathoanatomic characteristics of the nonunion must be assessed and a determination made about its etiology. The patient's regional and systemic comorbidities, soft tissue envelope, type of nonunion, and the presence or absence of a critical defect all factor into the surgeon's decision-making process. The treating surgeon must account for the initial injury mechanism, the extent of soft tissue stripping that may have occurred, and the resultant potential for devitalized bone. Laboratory studies to assess for possible endocrinopathies and nutritional deficiencies should be obtained.[12]

When considering the need for bone graft in the management of nonunions, the treating surgeon must have an in-depth understanding of the unique challenges presented by a given case. The treatment strategy for a hypertrophic femoral shaft nonunion in an otherwise healthy patient with an undersized intramedullary nail may not require autograft harvest and may be remedied with a simple exchange nailing. However, an atrophic distal tibial nonunion with a segmental defect and a draining sinus tract in a poor host may require multiple surgical efforts to achieve the goal of an aseptic union.

Once the surgeon has deemed autograft to be necessary in the treatment of a particular nonunion, he or she must select a graft harvest site. Among the described harvest sites for autogenous cancellous graft are anterior and posterior ICBG, distal femur, proximal tibia, and distal tibia. Takemoto and colleagues[13] compared messenger RNA levels of BMPs from various cancellous graft sites and found no significant difference between them. This would suggest that the osteogenic and osteoinductive properties are comparable between the tested cancellous beds. Conversely, Chiodo and colleagues[14] histologically examined iliac crest and proximal tibial cancellous bone and concluded that the iliac crest contained significantly more active hematopoietic marrow. Irrespective of their reported biochemical properties, many of these graft sites lack the volume required to address large bone defects.

Intramedullary bone graft harvest using the RIA consistently provides the quantities of bone graft required for addressing large bone defects and yields similar union rates when compared with ICBG. In a prospective study, McCall and colleagues[15] treated 20 bone defects ranging from 2.0 to 14.5 cm (average 6.6 cm) with RIA autograft. These investigators reported an average graft volume of 64 mL and achieved union in 17 (85%) of 20 patients. Dawson and colleagues[16] published a prospective randomized controlled study directly comparing ICBG to RIA for the treatment of nonunions. A total of 113 patients with nonunions underwent surgical repair with either ICBG (57) or RIA (56) and were followed until radiographic union. In addition to Short Musculoskeletal Functional Assessment and visual analogue scale scores, they collected operative data including graft volume harvested, time of harvest, and associated surgical costs. They concluded that RIA autograft achieves similar union rates (RIA, 82%; ICBG, 86%) with significantly less donor site pain. Furthermore, they noted that RIA was associated with shorter harvest times and was more cost-effective when accounting for the cost of increased operating room time when obtaining ICBG.

REAMER-IRRIGATOR-ASPIRATOR AND THE INDUCED MEMBRANE TECHNIQUE

In his original description of the induced membrane technique for management of segmental long bone defects, Masquelet and colleagues[17,18] reported successful union in 31 (89%) of 35 cases. They treated patients with defects ranging from 4 to 25 cm in a staged fashion. The described technique consists of first excision of devitalized or infected bone, the introduction of a polymethylmethacrylate (PMMA) cement spacer into the defect, and concurrent restoration of the soft tissue envelope. They posited that the cement spacer facilitated the formation of a pseudosynovial membrane and prevented soft tissue involution. Furthermore, the membrane functioned to prevent graft resorption and promote vascularity and corticalization. More recent studies to further define the role of the membrane have revealed that it is highly vascularized and secretes abundant growth factors, such as VEGF, transforming growth factor-β, and BMP-2. It has been additionally demonstrated that the membrane promotes osteogenic differentiation of MSCs.[19,20] The second stage consisted of atraumatic extraction of the PMMA spacer with preservation of the pseudosynovial membrane and autologous grafting with anterior ICBG. Interestingly, they noted that time to graft consolidation and subsequent union were independent of defect size.

Since it was initially described, the induced membrane technique has seen widespread application among traumatologists treating segmental long bone defects. Obremsky and

colleagues[21] conducted a survey of Orthopedic Trauma Association members regarding the management of these injuries. Overall, 89.5% (339 of 379) of respondents stated they used antibiotic cement spacers before the definitive bone-grafting procedure. It should be noted, however, that Masquelet himself discouraged the inclusion of antibiotics in the cement spacer due to potential adverse effects on the membrane and the possibility of suppressing without resolving infection. The elegant simplicity of the induced membrane technique has likely played a role in its popularity. It does not require the expertise of microvascular techniques nor the prolonged treatment times and patient burden of distraction osteogenesis and thus avoids the potential complications of both.[22]

With its rise in popularity, Masquelet's technique has seen expansion of indications. Originally described for treatment of bone loss resulting from septic nonunion, it has been successfully expanded to include segmental bone loss of any etiology. In addition, the technique has been successfully used with RIA autograft rather than ICBG.[15,23,24] Stafford and Norris[25] treated 27 bone defects ranging from 1 to 25 cm with the induced membrane technique and subsequent RIA autografting. They achieved clinical and radiographic union in 24 (89%) of 27 cases at 1 year. However, they did so with the inclusion of BMP in 23 (85%) of 27 cases.[25] In 2016, Morelli and colleagues[26] conducted a systematic review and meta-analysis of bony defects treated with the induced membrane technique. Seventeen studies met their inclusion criteria, with 427 patients undergoing treatment with the induced membrane technique. Of these, 137 (32%) were treated with RIA autograft. In the cohort of patients who received RIA, 116 of 137 went on to successful union.

CLINICAL CASES
Case 1
A 57-year-old otherwise healthy man who presented after a high-speed motorcycle collision with a displaced right femoral neck fracture, minimally displaced juxta-tectal transverse acetabular fracture, ipsilateral type 3A open AO/OTA 33.C3 distal femur with a 10 cm segmental defect and comminuted patellar fractures, contralateral both bone forearm and ipsilateral intra-articular distal radius fractures. He initially underwent irrigation and debridement of open fractures, open reduction and internal fixation (ORIF) of his femoral neck fracture, and application of knee-spanning external fixator. A few days later, he underwent ORIF of his patella

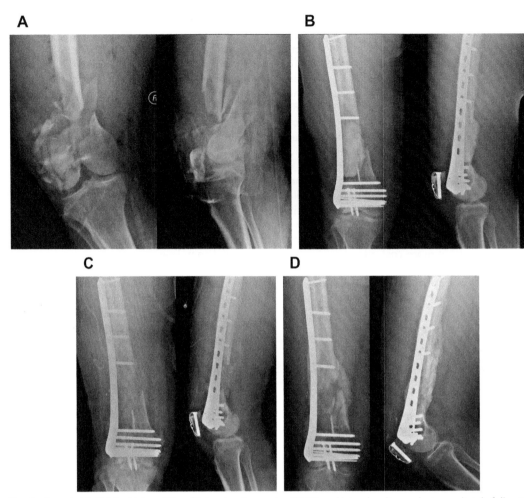

Fig. 1. Case 1. (*A*) Original injury AP and lateral radiographs. (*B*) AP and lateral radiographs immediately following ORIF and cement spacer placement. (*C*) AP and lateral radiographs immediately following RIA autograft. (*D*) AP and lateral radiographs 1 year after RIA autograft.

and distal femur fracture with inclusion of PMMA cement spacer with planned staged autologous bone grafting with induced membrane technique. He underwent extraction of his cement spacer and autograft with RIA obtained from the contralateral femur at 6 weeks. He remained toe touch weight bearing for a period of 12 weeks and went on to uncomplicated clinical and radiographic union. At 1-year follow-up, the patient complained of some persistent knee pain, but has been able to return to work in construction as a laborer (**Fig. 1**).

Case 2

A 28-year-old, otherwise healthy, right-hand-dominant man who was involved in a motor vehicle collision and sustained a grossly contaminated, left type 3A open 13.C3 distal humerus and 2U1C3 olecranon fractures with incomplete radial nerve palsy and traumatic bone loss resulting in an 8-cm segmental defect in addition to an intra-articular calcaneus fracture. The patient's left upper and lower extremity injuries were initially treated with irrigation and debridement, antibiotic bead placement, and spanning external fixation. Three days later, the patient was treated with ORIF of his humeral and ulnar fractures with placement of an antibiotic-impregnated PMMA cement spacer into the humeral meta-diaphyseal bone defect. Six weeks after definitive ORIF and spacer placement, the patient underwent removal of cement spacer and RIA autografting with the induced membrane technique. At 1-year post grafting, the patient had developed a humeral nonunion with hardware failure and new-onset ulnar nerve paresthesias. He underwent removal of hardware and nonunion repair with revision dual-column

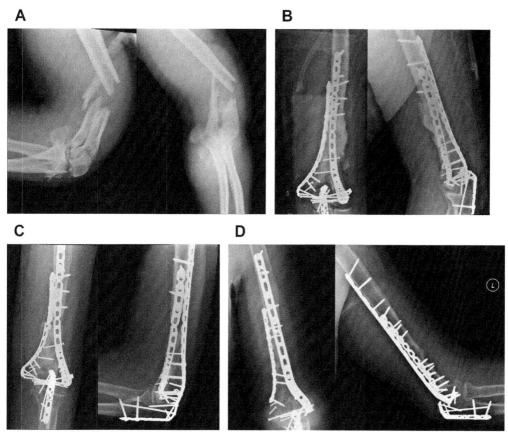

Fig. 2. Case 2. (*A*) Original injury AP and lateral radiographs. (*B*) AP and lateral radiographs immediately following ORIF and cement spacer placement. (*C*) AP and lateral radiographs 1 year after RIA autograft with nonunion and implant failure. (*D*) AP and lateral radiographs 1 year after nonunion repair with posterior ICBG.

plating. The patient was intentionally shortened by approximately 1 cm to create bony apposition and allow for compression plating. The nonunion repair was supplemented with cancellous posterior ICBG. He subsequently achieved aseptic union, and at 2-year follow-up reported no functional limitations with respect to his elbow, had full neurologic recovery, and demonstrated 30 to 120° of elbow motion. He did, however, report persistent hindfoot pain and demonstrated features of subtalar arthritis secondary to his calcaneus fracture, which had been treated with ORIF (Fig. 2).

Case 3

A healthy, 46-year-old man who was involved in an all-terrain vehicle crash and sustained a type 3B open distal meta-diaphyseal tibia fracture with a 3.5-cm intercalary bony defect and segmental distal fibula fracture. The patient was initially treated on the day of injury at an outside institution with irrigation and debridement, spanning external fixation, and a negative-pressure dressing. The patient was found to have an early wound infection on presentation to our facility and was initially treated with revision external fixation, serial repeat irrigation and debridement, and antibiotic bead placement. After apparent resolution of infection, the patient underwent ORIF of his segmental fibula fracture and reamed interlocked nailing of the tibia with PMMA spacer. Within 24 hours of definitive fixation, the patient underwent free tissue transfer with latissimus dorsl flap and skin grafting with retention of the transarticular external fixator to protect the flap. Although the initial plan was to delay grafting for 3 months to allow maturation of the flap, the patient's soft tissues and flap healing were delayed. At 5 months after definitive fixation of his tibia and fibular fractures, the patient underwent removal of antibiotic spacer and RIA autografting. He subsequently went on to uncomplicated union. At 1 year after his autograft procedure, the patient has not been able to return to work as a heavy laborer, is able to

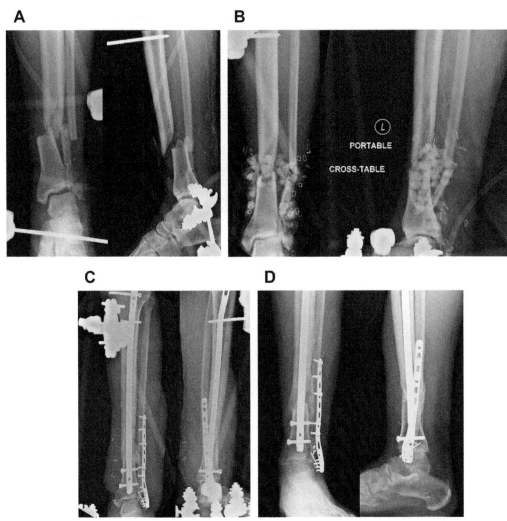

Fig. 3. Case 3. (*A*) AP and lateral radiographs on presentation to our institution. (*B*) AP and lateral radiographs after revision external fixation, irrigation and debridement, and antibiotic bead placement immediately following ORIF and cement spacer placement. (*C*) AP and lateral radiographs immediately following intramedullary nailing and cement spacer placement. (*D*) AP and lateral radiographs 1 year after RIA autograft.

walk unassisted with a leaf spring ankle foot orthosis, but has developed clinical and radiographic features of tibiotalar arthritis (**Fig. 3**).

REAMER-IRRIGATOR-ASPIRATOR AUTOGRAFT: PEARLS AND PITFALLS

As is the case with any surgical procedure, preoperative planning and well-executed surgical tactics are indispensable when using the RIA system to obtain autograft. Preoperative orthogonal imaging of the planned harvest bone should be obtained. Although the RIA system has proven to be generally safe, there are several somewhat predictable complications associated with its use:

1. Intraoperative blood loss and transfusions. Although blood loss is a less frequently discussed complication, the risk of significant blood loss in a short period of time exists. Several studies have noted this complication but, to our knowledge, only one has directly evaluated it. Marchand and colleagues[27] retrospectively reviewed 108 patients requiring bone graft harvest via RIA or ICBG and assessed the change in hematocrit (Hct) both preoperatively and postoperatively. The investigators concluded that RIA resulted in a decrease of Hct of 13.7 versus 7.36 with ICBG and that RIA patients were significantly more likely to require blood transfusions. They, however,

did not offer recommendations for mitigating this complication.

- Consider patient autotransfusion via technologies such as Cell Saver.
- Communication with the anesthesia team is paramount, particularly when treating patients with cardiovascular disease or otherwise diminished physiologic reserves.
- In addition, we recommend selecting a reamer head no larger than 1.5 mm larger than the narrowest portion of the femoral canal as measured on intraoperative fluoroscopy.
- Most importantly, if the reamer stalls or cannot easily pass due to excessively hard bone or reamer/canal size mismatch, we recommend extracting the reamer, downsizing, and sequentially reaming. Stalling the forward progress of the reamer while the suction remains connected will lead to rapid blood loss.
- Alternatively, if downsizing the reamer head is not an option, we recommend temporarily clamping the suction.

2. Cortical Perforation and Eccentric Reaming
- As is the case with intramedullary nailing, particular attention must be paid to starting point and opening reamer trajectories. In the femur, piriformis, trochanteric, and retrograde RIA harvests are well described.[28] We prefer the use of a piriformis starting point to minimize the entry angle of the reamer. Particularly in patients with Dorr A femoral canals, a lateral entry starting point that is not in line with the axis of the canal may predispose to stalling and eccentric reaming of the medial cortex.
- Care should be taken regarding the position of the guidewire within the distal femur to ensure it is not resting on the anterior cortex in the supracondylar region.

3. Donor Site Fracture
- Again, we advise against reaming diameters greater than 1.5 mm beyond the narrowest portion of the isthmus. Rather than increasing to 2 mm, redirecting the guidewire into the medial and lateral condyles of the femur will augment graft volume. However, a very tight distal bend in the guidewire may result in unplanned advancement of the guidewire if the bend does not allow unimpeded progress of the RIA.
- When using the ossimeter and intraoperative fluoroscopy, it is important to remember that measurement of canal diameter will be affected as the ruler's distance from the bone changes as a result of image intensifier magnification. This may become more relevant when treating obese patients. In an obese patient, the distance between the bone and ossimeter is increased when compared with a thin patient. Placing the ossimeter over the anterior thigh in the anteroposterior (AP) projection with the receiver above the patient will cause the canal to appear larger and the ossimeter to appear smaller. This may lead to selection of a larger reaming head than is appropriate. This projectional illusion may be accounted for with the following:
  o A distance of 25 mm between the ossimeter and bone will yield a measurement that appears fluoroscopically to be 1 mm larger than actual canal diameter
  o 50 mm = measurement 2 mm larger than canal
  o 100 mm = measurement 3 mm larger than canal

SUMMARY

The RIA autograft was initially designed to address the problems of fat embolism and thermal necrosis, which had previously been unsolved and have plagued clinicians since the 1940s. However, the simple addition of an inline filter and collection device allowed surgeons to efficiently take advantage of the intramedullary canal as a source of autograft. RIA autograft provides large volumes of autogenous graft that have been shown to exhibit excellent osteogenic, osteoinductive, and osteoconductive properties. These features, combined with the relative ease of graft harvest and low donor site morbidity when compared with the gold standard ICBG, have made RIA autograft, at the very least, a viable alternative to ICBG. Some would suggest RIA autograft to be superior to ICBG, particularly in the setting of large segmental bone defects managed with the induced membrane technique. And although significant complications such as fracture and cortical perforation have been reported, they are preventable if proper surgical strategy and tactics are used.

REFERENCES

1. Vecsei V, Hajdu S, Negrin LL. Intramedullary nailing in fracture treatment: history, science and Kuntscher's revolutionary influence in Vienna, Austria. Injury 2011;42(Suppl 4):S1–5.

2. Danckwardt-Lilliestrom G, Lorenzi L, Olerud S. Intracortical circulation after intramedullary reaming with reduction of pressure in the medullary cavity. J Bone Joint Surg Am 1970;52(7):1390–4.

3. Green J. History and development of suction-irrigation-reaming. Injury 2010;41(Suppl 2):S24–31.

4. Johnson EE, Marder RA. Open intramedullary nailing and bone-grafting for non-union of tibial diaphyseal fracture. J Bone Joint Surg Am 1987;69(3):375–80.

5. Haubruck P, Ober J, Heller R, et al. Complications and risk management in the use of the reaming-irrigator-aspirator (RIA) system: RIA is a safe and reliable method in harvesting autologous bone graft. PLoS One 2018;13(4):e0196051.

6. Ahlmann E, Patzakis M, Roidis N, et al. Comparison of anterior and posterior iliac crest bone grafts in terms of harvest-site morbidity and functional outcomes. J Bone Joint Surg Am 2002;84-A(5):716–20.

7. Fowler BL, Dall BE, Rowe DE. Complications associated with harvesting autogenous iliac bone graft. Am J Orthop (Belle Mead NJ) 1995;24(12):895–903.

8. Frolke JP, Nulend JK, Semeins CM, et al. Viable osteoblastic potential of cortical reamings from intramedullary nailing. J Orthop Res 2004;22(6):1271–5.

9. Schmidmaier G, Herrmann S, Green J, et al. Quantitative assessment of growth factors in reaming aspirate, iliac crest, and platelet preparation. Bone 2006;39(5):1156–63.

10. Yin T, Li L. The stem cell niches in bone. J Clin Invest 2006;116(5):1195–201.

11. Sagi HC, Young ML, Gerstenfeld L, et al. Qualitative and quantitative differences between bone graft obtained from the medullary canal (with a Reamer/Irrigator/Aspirator) and the iliac crest of the same patient. J Bone Joint Surg Am 2012; 94(23):2128–35.

12. Brinker MR, O'Connor DP, Monla YT, et al. Metabolic and endocrine abnormalities in patients with nonunions. J Orthop Trauma 2007;21(8):557–70.

13. Takemoto RC, Fajardo M, Kirsch T, et al. Quantitative assessment of the bone morphogenetic protein expression from alternate bone graft harvesting sites. J Orthop Trauma 2010;24(9):564–6.

14. Chiodo CP, Hahne J, Wilson MG, et al. Histological differences in iliac and tibial bone graft. Foot Ankle Int 2010;31(5):418–22.

15. McCall TA, Brokaw DS, Jelen BA, et al. Treatment of large segmental bone defects with Reamer-Irrigator-Aspirator bone graft: technique and case series. Orthop Clin North Am 2010;41(1):63–73. table of contents.

16. Dawson J, Kiner D, Gardner W 2nd, et al. The Reamer-Irrigator-Aspirator as a device for harvesting bone graft compared with iliac crest bone graft: union rates and complications. J Orthop Trauma 2014;28(10):584–90.

17. Masquelet AC, Fitoussi F, Begue T, et al. Reconstruction of the long bones by the induced membrane and spongy autograft. Ann Chir Plast Esthet 2000;45(3):346–53 [in French].

18. Masquelet AC. Muscle reconstruction in reconstructive surgery: soft tissue repair and long bone reconstruction. Langenbecks Arch Surg 2003; 388(5):344–6.

19. Gruber HE, Ode G, Hoelscher G, et al. Osteogenic, stem cell and molecular characterisation of the human induced membrane from extremity bone defects. Bone Joint Res 2016;5(4):106–15.

20. Pelissier P, Masquelet AC, Bareille R, et al. Induced membranes secrete growth factors including vascular and osteoinductive factors and could stimulate bone regeneration. J Orthop Res 2004;22(1): 73–9.

21. Obremskey W, Molina C, Collinge C, et al. Current practice in the management of open fractures among orthopaedic trauma surgeons. Part B: management of segmental long bone defects. a survey of orthopaedic trauma association members. J Orthop Trauma 2014;28(8):e203–7.

22. Masquelet AC. Induced membrane technique: pearls and pitfalls. J Orthop Trauma 2017; 31(Suppl 5):S36–8.

23. Apard T, Bigorre N, Cronier P, et al. Two-stage reconstruction of post-traumatic segmental tibia bone loss with nailing. Orthop Traumatol Surg Res 2010;96(5):549–53.

24. Huffman LK, Harris JG, Suk M. Using the bi-Masquelet technique and Reamer-Irrigator-Aspirator for post-traumatic foot reconstruction. Foot Ankle Int 2009;30(9):895–9.

25. Stafford PR, Norris BL. Reamer-Irrigator-Aspirator bone graft and bi Masquelet technique for segmental bone defect nonunions: a review of 25 cases. Injury 2010;41(Suppl 2):S72–7.

26. Morelli I, Drago L, George DA, et al. Masquelet technique: myth or reality? A systematic review and meta-analysis. Injury 2016;47(Suppl 6):S68–76.

27. Marchand LS, Rothberg DL, Kubiak EN, et al. Is this autograft worth it? The blood loss and transfusion rates associated with reamer irrigator aspirator bone graft harvest. J Orthop Trauma 2017;31(4):205–9.

28. Finnan RP, Prayson MJ, Goswami T, et al. Use of the Reamer-Irrigator-Aspirator for bone graft harvest: a mechanical comparison of three starting points in cadaveric femurs. J Orthop Trauma 2010;24(1): 36–41.

Arthroscopic-Assisted Reduction of Tibial Plateau Fractures

Rebecca Chase, DO[b], Kudret Usmani, MD[a],*,
Alisina Shahi, MD[a], Kenneth Graf, MD[a],
Rakesh Mashru, MD[a]

KEYWORDS

- Arthroscopic reduction • Tibial plateau fractures • Classification • Indications
- Contraindications • Surgical technique • Complications • Outcomes • Schatzker classification

---

KEY POINTS

- Arthroscopic reduction of tibial plateau fractures has been gaining in popularity, with advantages including accurate diagnosis and treatment, minimally invasive dissection, quicker recovery, and anatomic reduction of joint surface.
- The success of arthroscopic reduction depends on accurate fracture selection, with Schatzker fracture patterns I, II and III benefitting the most from effective arthroscopic-assisted reduction techniques.
- With arthroscopic-assisted reduction of tibial plateau fractures, patient set-up is similar to standard knee arthroscopy, but the C-arm is used to help with fracture reduction and fixation.
- Outcomes of arthroscopic-assisted reduction are promising with multiple studies demonstrating equivalent knee outcome scores.

INTRODUCTION: NATURE OF THE PROBLEM

Fractures of the tibial plateau comprise around 1% of all fractures, but can represent significant morbidity for patients and a significant challenge for many orthopedic surgeons.[1] Fractures of the tibial plateau involve the articular surface and the metaphysis of the proximal tibia. These fractures tend to have a bimodal age distribution, often occurring in young adults with high-energy trauma such as motor vehicle collisions and in the elderly with osteoporotic bone, who sustain these fractures from low-impact trauma such as falls from standing height.[2] Tibial plateau fractures have a variety of fracture patterns and a multitude of treatment options, including cast immobilization, skeletal traction, external fixation, and open reduction internal fixation.[2] Surgical management can be challenging, with the main goals of treatment defined as obtaining anatomic reduction of the articular surface, satisfactory alignment, stable fixation allowing early mobilization, and minimal soft tissue injury.[3] With the recent trend toward minimally invasive techniques, arthroscopic-assisted fracture reduction and fixation has been gaining interest in the orthopedic community.

Tibial plateau fractures are commonly associated with significant soft tissue injuries. The incidence of soft tissue injury with tibial plateau fractures that can be addressed during arthroscopy has been shown to be as high as 71%, with injury to the meniscus in 57%, anterior cruciate ligament (ACL) in 25%, posterior cruciate ligament in 5%, lateral collateral ligament in

---

Disclosure Statement: The authors have nothing to disclose.

[a] Cooper University Hospital, Three Cooper Plaza, Suite 408, Camden, NJ 08103, USA; [b] Philadelphia College of Osteopathic Medicine, 4190 City Avenue, Suite 320, Philadelphia, PA 19131, USA

* Corresponding author.

E-mail address: usmani-kudret@cooperhealth.edu

3%, and medial collateral ligament in 3%.[2] Arthroscopy can range from just a diagnostic examination, debridement, and partial meniscectomy, to arthroscopic reduction and internal fixation with bone grafting. Advantages of arthroscopy include an accurate diagnosis and treatment of joint pathology, less soft tissue dissection, no requirement for a formal arthrotomy or detachment of the anterior horn of the lateral meniscus, better and faster recovery of joint motion, and anatomic restoration of the joint surface.[4,5] Some disadvantages of arthroscopic-assisted reduction include longer operative times, fluid extravasation into the operative limb, higher cost of the procedure, and the potential for less rigid fixation with percutaneous techniques.[2,4] The most critical factor in deciding when to use arthroscopic-assisted treatment is appropriate fracture selection, but do the benefits outweigh the risks, and is this a technique worth investing time in perfecting?

CLASSIFICATION

Although there are many classification systems for tibial plateau fractures, the 2 most commonly used classification systems are the Schatzker and the OTA/AO classification systems.[6] Based on the Schatzker classification, fractures are classified based on degree of articular involvement with increasing Schatzker type correlating with increasing order of severity and instability. Type I is a pure split of the lateral plateau as a result of a valgus and axial force that is often seen in younger patients. Type II is a split fracture of the lateral plateau with an associated depression. The mechanism is similar to type I, with either a greater force or weaker bone quality. Type III is a pure depression fracture of the lateral plateau as a result of an axial force. Type IV is a fracture of the medial tibial plateau with a varus or axial directed force. The force

needed to cause medial tibial plateau fractures is generally greater than the force seen with type I, II, or III fractures. Type V is a fracture of both the lateral and medial condyles. Type IV is a bicondylar fracture with metaphyseal–diaphyseal dissociation.[2,6]

The OTA/OA classification system classifies tibial plateau fractures as 41B or 41C depending on whether the fracture has partial articular or complete articular surface involvement. The 41B1 fractures involve a unicondylar split fracture, 41B2 involve a unicondylar depression fracture, and 41B3 involve a split depression-type fracture pattern of the medial or lateral tibial plateaus. The 41C fracture patterns define fracture patterns that involve the articular and metaphyseal proximal tibia, with 41C1 defined as simple articular, simple metaphyseal fractures, 41C2 defined as simple articular wedge or multifragmentary metaphyseal fractures, and 41C3 as fragmentary or multifragmentary metaphyseal fractures.[7,8]

INDICATIONS AND CONTRAINDICATIONS

Reports have shown that arthroscopic-assisted techniques can be more effective in Schatzker types I, II, and III fractures compared with more complex fracture patterns. Unicondylar fractures tend to show better results than bicondylar fractures.[4] During arthroscopic procedures, if the cortical envelop cannot be easily restored, then open techniques are prudent. Comminuted fractures and Schatzker types IV to VI are generally not recommended for treatment with arthroscopic techniques because of increased risk of fluid extravasation, which could lead to a compartment syndrome (Table 1).[4]

SURGICAL TECHNIQUE
Preoperative Planning
Surgical technique is usually dictated by the fracture pattern. The anteroposterior and lateral

Table 1		
Indications and contraindications for using arthroscopy with tibial plateau fracture fixation		
	Indications	**Contraindications**
Arthroscopic-assisted tibial plateau reductions	Schatzker I, II, or III fracture patterns Preoperative MRI demonstrating known meniscus or ligament tear that needs to be addressed Significant soft tissue injury that would benefit from less invasive techniques Direct visualization of the joint reduction along with fluoroscopy	Significantly comminuted Schatzker IV, V, or VI fracture patterns Complex fracture patterns where the cortical window cannot easily be restored Any patient with preexisting degenerative joint disease

radiographs of the knee should be scrutinized to evaluate the fracture pattern and to rule out concomitant injuries.[3,4] To fully understand the fracture pattern, a computed tomography scan is critical and can help to better assess the cortical envelope. The cortical envelope refers to the outer rim of the plateau and in most Schatzker I through III fractures is still intact or can be easily reduced with a clamp.[9] An MRI can also be used in an acute setting to detect concomitant soft tissue injuries. Meniscus and ACL injuries have been observed as the most common combined soft tissue injuries and may be treated with arthroscopic-assisted fixation at the time of the initial surgery.[6]

Preparation and Patient Positioning

The patient set-up is similar to a standard knee arthroscopy with the patient supine on the operating room table. The affected leg can be placed in a leg holder. However, the holder should be positioned slightly more proximal than the usual setting to allow more room for the C-arm. Verify before the leg is prepped and draped that images can be obtained. Other ways to position the leg include using a lateral post at the proximal thigh, away from the fracture site, and placing the foot on a paint roller. The paint roller is present for the foot to be wedged allowing the knee to be placed in flexion. Alternatively, the paint roller can be used as a post under the thigh to allow the lower leg to hang off the side of the table.[5,10] A nonsterile or sterile tourniquet can be used and a sterile U drape with access to the ipsilateral iliac crest can be considered if iliac crest bone harvest is to be used for bone grafting instead of allograft or other augments.[6] The C-arm can be positioned on the contralateral side and monitors for fluoroscopy and arthroscopy can be placed on the ipsilateral side for best visualization of the joint and unobstructed anteroposterior and lateral images during the case. The fluoroscopy monitor can also be set at the base of the patient table if preferred for viewing (**Fig. 1**). The general equipment needed is a 2.7-mm guide pin and aiming arm from an ACL set, rigid 10- to 11-mm cannulated reamers, partially threaded cannulated screws and washers, bone graft, cannulated versus solid tamps, and reduction clamps and other tools needed to aid in reduction.

SURGICAL APPROACH

Similar to a standard knee arthroscopic technique, an anterolateral portal is made and the arthroscope is introduced into the joint. An anteromedial portal is made under direct visualization to use for instrument introduction. Owing to the increased concern for fluid extravasation and compartment syndrome, irrigation of the knee should be done with gravity for the fluid inflow.[11] If a pressure pump is going to be used, it should not be set higher than 40 to 50 mm Hg and compartment firmness should be checked throughout the procedure.[4,6] A third portal in the superior lateral position can be used to help evacuate fracture hematoma and maintain low joint pressures.

SURGICAL PROCEDURE

The first step in arthroscopic reduction internal fixation techniques is to obtain direct visualization of the joint, which can be complicated by significant fracture hematoma. The joint should be irrigated to evacuate the fracture hematoma and improve visibility. Upon obtaining sufficient visibility, a full diagnostic evaluation is performed to identify bone and cartilage lesions as well as damage to menisci, ACL, or posterior cruciate ligament[10] (**Fig. 2**). If the fracture is located more lateral and is underneath the meniscus, a loop around the meniscus can be placed to lift it out of the way or meniscus hooks can be used for retraction to expose the fracture.[6]

Fractures with a split component can be reduced with a clamp, using a spatula or probe to help elevate the fragment and reconstitute a level joint surface. One or 2 K-wires can also be inserted into the fractured plateau and used as joysticks to manipulate to the fragment.[6] After checking the reduction with both fluoroscopy and arthroscopy, the fracture fragment can be temporarily held with K-wires parallel to and about 1 cm distal to the joint line.[6]

Depressed fracture patterns require elevation of the articular surface attached to the fracture fragment, and articular reduction depends on the application of an elevating force at the center of the depression. ACL aiming systems can facilitate the accurate insertion of a guide pin into the center of the depression.[6,11,12] The guide pin can be inserted through the damaged condyle or the intact condyle. Although going through the intact condyle allows for a larger volume of cancellous bone to support the subchondral bone, the tamp used to elevate the joint surface is coming from a more tangential direction and risks causing damage to the intact condyle. Once adequate positioning of the guide pin is achieved a 2- to 3-cm incision is

A

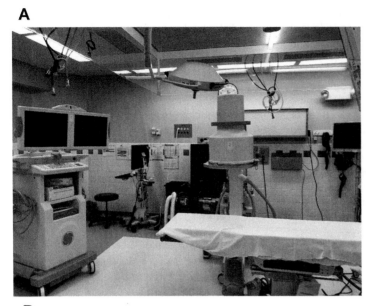

B

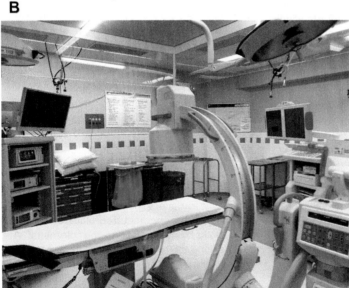

Fig. 1. (*A*, *B*) Room setup if the tibial plateau fracture was on the left leg: C-arm on the contralateral side, arthroscopy monitor/tower on the ipsilateral side, and fluoroscopy monitor at the bottom of the bed.

made around the guide pin and is dissected down to bone. An anterior cortical window is created with a cannulated reamer about 10 to 11 mm in diameter 1 to 2 cm below the depression.[6,13] If a cannulated tamp or impactor is available, the guide pin can be left in place and bone graft gently tamped in below the depression to elevate the joint surface. The use of cannulated tamps with an angulated surface allows the elevation of the depressed surface perpendicular to the joint surface. Fluoroscopic and arthroscopic imaging should be monitored while impacting the bone graft with the goal of slight overcorrection of the joint surface. Then, during knee flexion and extension, the femoral

condyle articulation with the tibial joint surface can be used to mold the tibial joint surface.[6] The elevated surface can be temporarily held with K-wires about 1 cm below the joint surface. Another technique uses intraosseous balloon-assisted repositioning of the depressed tibial plateau fracture with an injection of calcium phosphate cement in a liquid or paste form using arthroscopy and fluoroscopy to aid in evaluating anatomic alignment and to verify no cement escapes.[14]

Using 2 or 3 large diameter cannulated screws parallel to the joint surface placed percutaneously with washers is an acceptable fixation method for lateral tibial plateau fractures.[15] If

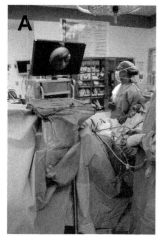
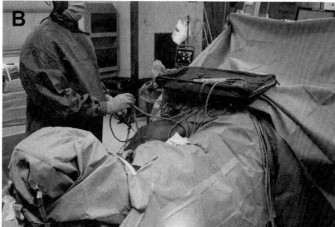
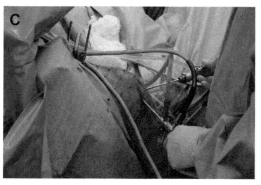
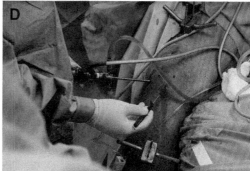

Fig. 2. (A–D) Example of arthroscopy performed for a patient with tibial plateau fracture. Notice the knee-spanning external fixator pins in place.

fracture instability is a concern, a buttress screw can be placed percutaneously at the inferior apex of the split fragment. A buttress plate can also be placed through submuscular techniques or through traditional extraarticular incisions.[2]

COMPLEX TIBIAL PLATEAU FRACTURES

Schatzker type V and VI fractures are commonly the result of high-energy injuries with significant comminution, soft tissue injury, and articular step off. These types of fractures normally require open reduction and bilateral buttress plating, and are not amenable to percutaneous screw fixation as a stable construct for fracture fixation. Some surgeons believe arthroscopic-assisted reduction with bilateral buttress plate fixation offers a good alternative to large open arthrotomy incision required with open reduction internal fixation. The set-up is the same as for arthroscopically treating Schatzker types I through III, and the reduction technique is similar with ACL tibial guides being used to localize the center of the depression and K-wires as joysticks to reduce the split components. Skin

incisions are made medial and lateral to fit the buttress plates and care is taken to avoid an arthrotomy. In a study of 18 patients treated with this technique by Chan and colleagues,[3] all 18 fractures united; 4 patients were rated as excellent, 12 as good, and 2 as fair for overall results at an average of 48 months of follow-up. Fig. 3 provides an algorithm for arthroscopic-assisted treatment of tibial plateau fractures based on fracture pattern.

TREATMENT OF SOFT TISSUES

Meniscal lesions that are amenable to suture repair can be repaired with conventional arthroscopic methods. Partial meniscectomy is done when the meniscus tear is not indicated for suture repair. The knee should be examined before and after fixation with stress radiographs to evaluate the integrity of the collateral ligaments. Although most collateral ligament lesions can be managed conservatively, significant medial and/or lateral laxity may require surgical ligamentous repair. Although ACL tears are common with tibial plateau fractures, most are

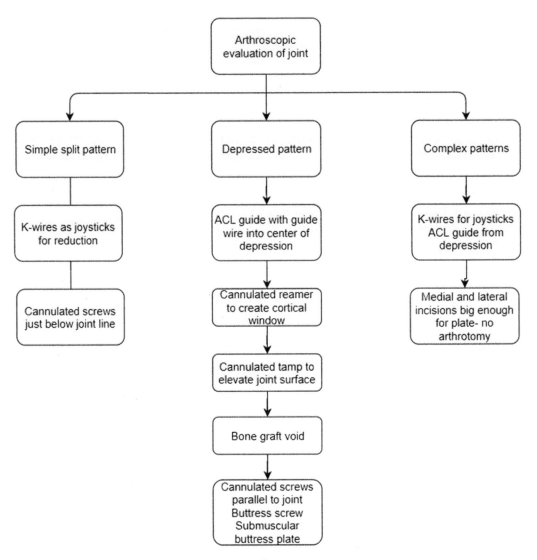

Fig. 3. Flow chart of treatment options depending on fracture pattern.

asymptomatic and can be observed after fracture fixation. If a concomitant ACL tear is found to be associated with chronic knee instability, a staged secondary procedure for ACL reconstruction can be done at a later date.[13] The only cruciate ligament injuries amenable to repair at the time of arthroscopic-assisted fracture fixation are those caused by bony avulsion of the tibial footprint.[2]

POSTOPERATIVE CARE

The patient should be closely monitored in the acute postoperative period for compartment syndrome. Deep vein thrombosis prophylaxis should be started and continued while the patient is non-weight bearing, typically for 6 to

12 weeks. The patient can be placed in a hinged knee brace and gentle passive and active range of motion can be started.[5] A continuous passive motion machine can be used with initial settings starting around 0° to 60° and increasing the settings daily as tolerated.[15] Full weight bearing is usually delayed until 10 to 12 weeks postoperatively, but depending on the fracture pattern, achieved fixation, and radiographic evidence of healing, partial or foot-flat weight bearing can be started as early as 4 to 6 weeks after surgery.

COMPLICATIONS

Compartment syndrome is the most feared complication with arthroscopically assisted reductions owing to fluid extravasation. Keeping the pump pressure at less than 50 mm Hg makes this complication very rare.[6] Infection, wound complications, and thromboembolism are less commonly seen with arthroscopic reductions when compared with standard open repair techniques.[3,4]

CASE

A 26-year-old man lost control of his motorized off-road bicycle during a 20-foot jump and landed on his left leg. He had immediate pain in his left knee and was unable to ambulate or move his knee. In the trauma bay, he was noted to have a large effusion of his left knee and varus instability. His initial radiographs and computed tomography scan (Fig. 4) showed a depressed medial tibial plateau fracture with incongruence of his joint space. An MRI was obtained (Fig. 5) that revealed a depressed medial tibial condyle, with possible ACL and medial meniscus tear and an lateral collateral ligament tear. He underwent an arthroscopic-assisted open reduction internal fixation of his medial tibial plateau. After obtaining an anterolateral portal a 3-compartment diagnostic examination was completed, which demonstrated the depressed fracture of the medial tibial plateau (Fig. 6A). An anteromedial portal was made to introduce tools and his medial meniscus was closely examined with a probe and no tear was identified. A stress examination of his ACL and posterior cruciate ligament demonstrated no tears or obvious signs of subluxation. After cleaning the hemarthrosis, the fluid was evacuated and a 10-cm anteromedial incision was made over the proximal tibial plateau. Using osteotomes, curettes, and a freer elevator, the joint was elevated and reduced. This process was confirmed by fluoroscopic imaging. The arthroscope was then reinserted into the knee and confirmed the reduction of the joint surface. After confirming no articular step off of the joint arthroscopically (Fig. 6B), a medial to lateral rafting screw was placed before affixing the medial tibial plateau plate. Calcium phosphate cement was also used to buttress the depressed plateau. Intraoperative arthroscopic images demonstrated the improvement in his articular surface and restoration of joint congruence and no meniscus or ACL injuries. Postoperative radiographs confirmed anatomic reduction with restoration of the mechanical axis of his lower extremity (Fig. 7).

RESULTS REVIEW AND OUTCOMES

Fowble and colleagues[16] in a retrospective cohort compared arthroscopic treatment with traditional open techniques, with 12 patients treated by arthroscopic-assisted reduction and 11 open techniques. Overall the results for arthroscopic reduction were superior to open reduction internal fixation. In the arthroscopic group, all reductions were anatomic and remained fixed for at least 3 months, whereas only 6 (55%) of the open reduction internal fixation patients had anatomic reductions initially and 1 patient had subsequent further loss of reduction at follow-up. The average length of hospitalization for arthroscopic reduction patients was 5.36 days compared with 10.27 days for open reduction internal fixation. The average time to weight bearing was 8.95 weeks in the arthroscopic group and 12.30 weeks in the open group.[16]

Ohdera and colleagues[4] compared 28 patients treated arthroscopically or open and showed no statistical difference between the groups in terms of duration of operation, postoperative flexion, and clinical results. In the arthroscopic group, the postoperative rehabilitation was easier and faster with time to obtain

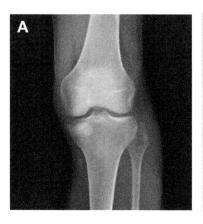
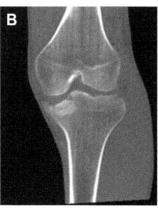

Fig. 4. (A) Initial injury anteroposterior radiograph of the left knee and (B) coronal cut of the injury computed tomography scan done showing a medial depressed tibial plateau fracture.

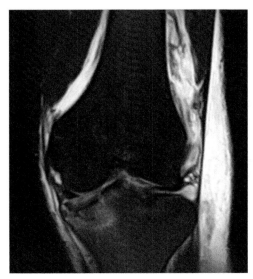

Fig. 5. MRI T2 coronal cut of left knee medial tibial plateau fracture.

fixation and open reduction internal fixation treatment for Schatzker type I fractures. Arthroscopic reduction and internal fixation may improve the clinical outcome in Schatzker type II, III, and IV fractures. In Schatzker types V and VI fractures, both techniques had poor medium- and long-term results, but arthroscopic reduction and internal fixation treatment, when indicated, is the best choice for lower rates of infection.[16]

Scheerlinck and colleagues obtained excellent HSS knee scores in 79% of patients with more than 5 years of follow-up. Scheerlinck and colleagues[19] also showed a return to the previous level of sporting activities in 63% of patients.

A study looking at the anatomic results of arthroscopically treated tibial plateau fractures with percutaneous osteosynthesis showed that the anatomic results were not modified and that the long-term results are as good as those fractures treated open for types III and IV. Cassard and colleagues[20] had 26 patients with 2 type I, 17 type II, 6 type III, and 1 type IV fractures were reduced arthroscopically and the fixation devices used were percutaneous cannulated screws in 23 cases, K-wires in 2 cases, and bone cement filing of the fracture site in 1 case.[18]

flexion of 120° at 4.6 weeks compared with 9.1 weeks for the open group. Eighty-four percent of the patients in the arthroscopic group obtained anatomic reduction, defined as less than 2 mm displacement, compared with only 55% of the patients in the open group.

Chan and colleagues[17] had a 2- to 10-year prospective follow-up study of 54 patients treated with arthroscopic-assisted reduction; good or excellent clinical and radiographic results were achieved in 96%. Secondary osteoarthritis was seen in 10 injured knees (19%). All 54 fractures successfully united, and no complications directly associated with arthroscopically were noted in any patients.

Dall'Oca and colleagues[18] compared arthroscopic-assisted reduction with open reduction and internal fixation with 12 to 116 month follow-up. They found that there was no difference in arthroscopic reduction and internal

Krause and colleagues[1] analyzed the anatomic reduction of complex tibial plateau fractures reduced and evaluated with fluoroscopy and then reevaluated with arthroscopy. Seven of 17 patients had satisfactory reduction with just fluoroscopy and 10 of the 17 had persistent depression seen arthroscopically that needed intraoperative correction. The cases that needed arthroscopic-assisted reduction had larger preoperative depression and fracture gap and it was also noted that arthroscopy helped with posterolaterocentral fragments as was confirmed on postoperative computed tomography.[19]

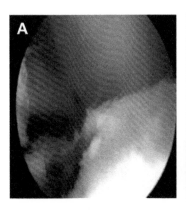
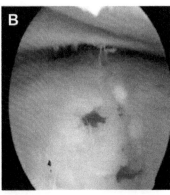

Fig. 6. Intraoperative arthroscopic images showing (A) the initial displacement and depression of the fracture and then (B) the joint surface after reduction.

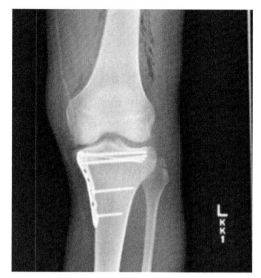

Fig. 7. Postoperative anteroposterior radiograph of left knee with reduction of the fracture and congruence of the joint surface.

SUMMARY

Arthroscopy can be a helpful aid to better evaluate and diagnose fracture patterns and assist in treatment of tibial plateau fixations especially for Schatzker types I to III patterns. Also, owing to the decreased amount of dissection needed with arthroscopically assisted reductions, this technique is being evaluated for more complex fracture patterns. Studies have shown that arthroscopic-assisted reduction is an effective technique with results showing the majority of patients having satisfactory clinical and radiological Rasmussen scores. Arthroscopy allows a more accurate evaluation of the fracture reduction and allows optimal treatment of concomitant lesions without having to make an extensive arthrotomy incision. Arthroscopic-assisted reduction has also been associated with decreased length of hospital stays and shorter postoperative rehabilitation time. Some disadvantages of this technique are higher cost and longer duration of the procedure. Also, the possibility of less rigid fixation then with plates needs to be further tested with biomechanical and clinical studies. There is a learning curve element with this technique, as with any other new surgical technique. Surgeon experience and fracture pattern play a very important role with the success rate of this procedure. Not all tibial plateau fracture patterns are ideal for arthroscopic-assisted reduction, but when it can be applied it is a useful tool for assessing at the joint reduction during surgery.

REFERENCES

1. Krause M, Preiss A, Meenen NM, et al. "Fracturoscopy" is superior to fluoroscopy in the articular reconstruction of complex tibial plateau fractures-an arthroscopy assisted fracture reduction technique. J Orthop Trauma 2016;30:437–44.
2. Lubowitz JH, Elson WS, Guttmann D, et al. Part I arthroscopic management of tibial plateau fractures. Arthroscopy 2004;20:1063–70.
3. Chen X-Z, Liu CG, Chen Y, et al. Arthroscopy-assisted surgery for tibial plateau fractures. Arthroscopy 2015;31(1):143–53.
4. Ohdera T, Tokunaga M, Hiroshima S, et al. Arthroscopic management of tibial plateau fractures-comparison with open reduction method. Arch Orthop Trauma Surg 2003;123:489–93.
5. Kiefer H, Zivaljevic N, Imbriglia JE, et al. Arthroscopic reduction and internal fixation (ARIF) of lateral tibial plateau fractures. Knee Surg Sports Traumatol Arthrosc 2001;9:167–72.
6. Burdin G. Arthroscopic management of tibial plateau fractures: surgical technique. Orthop Traumatol Surg Res 2013;99S:S208–18.
7. Meinberg E, Agel J, Roberts C, et al. Fracture and dislocation classification compendium–2018. J Orthop Trauma 2018;32(Suppl 1):S1–170.
8. Prat-Fabregat S, Camacho-Carrasco P. Treatment strategy for tibial plateau fractures: an update. EFORT Open Rev 2016;1(5):225–32.
9. Abdel-Hamid MZ, Chang CH, Chan YS, et al. Arthroscopic evaluation of soft tissue injuries in tibial plateau fractures: retrospective analysis of 98 cases. Arthroscopy 2006;22:669–75.
10. Hartigan DE, McCarthy MA, Krych AJ, et al. Arthroscopic-assisted reduction and percutaneous fixation of tibial plateau fractures. Arthrosc Tech 2015;4:e51–5.
11. Chan Y-S. Arthroscopy-assisted surgery for tibial plateau fractures. Chang Gung Med J 2011;34:239–47.
12. Suganuma J, Akutsu S. Arthroscopically assisted treatment of tibial plateau fractures. Arthroscopy 2004;20:1084–9.
13. Levy BA, Herrera DA, Macdonald P, et al. The "medial approach" for arthroscopic- assisted fixation of the lateral tibial plateau fractures: patient selection and mid-to long- term results. J Orthop Trauma 2008;22:201–5.
14. Ziogas K, et al. Arthroscopically assisted balloon osteoplasty of a tibial plateau depression fracture: a case report. N Am J Med Sci 2015;7:411–4.
15. Rossi R, Castoldi F, Blonna D, et al. Arthroscopic treatment of lateral tibial plateau fractures: a simple technique. Arthroscopy 2006;22:678.e1–6.
16. Fowble CD, Zimmer JW, Schepsis AA, et al. The role of arthroscopy in the assessment and treatment of tibial plateau fractures. Arthroscopy 1993;9:584–90.

17. Chan Y-S, Chiu CH, Lo YP, et al. Arthroscopy-assisted surgery for tibial plateau fractures: 2- to 10- year follow-up results. Arthroscopy 2008;24: 760–8.

18. Dall'Oca C, Maluta T, Lavini F, et al. Tibial plateau fractures: compared between ARIF and ORIF. Strategies Trauma Limb Reconstr 2012;7: 163–75.

19. Scheerlinck t, Ng CS, Handelberg F, et al. Medium-term results of percutaneous, arthroscopically-assisted, osteosynthesis of fractures of the tibial plateau. J Bone Joint Surg Br 1998;80:959–64.

20. Cassard X, Beaufils P, Blin JL, et al. Osteosynthesis under arthroscopic control of separated tibial plateau fractures. 26 case reports. Rev Chir Orthop Reparatrice Appar Mot 1999;85:257–66.

Pediatrics

Pediatric Orthopedic Workforce

A Review of Recent Trends

Arya Minaie, BA[a], Maksim A. Shlykov, MD, MS[a],
Pooya Hosseinzadeh, MD[b,*]

KEYWORDS

• Pediatric orthopedic surgery • POSNA • Sports medicine • Workforce

KEY POINTS

- The field of pediatric orthopedic surgery has seen massive growth in both applicants and fellowship positions over the past 2 decades.
- Pediatric orthopedic surgery continues to lead the way in gender diversity in orthopedics.
- Caseload data suggest that new pediatric orthopedic subspecialties may be emerging.
- Although more pediatric surgeons are being trained annually, competition does not currently appear to be an issue due to retiring surgeons and increased total case volume.

INTRODUCTION

An overall trend toward specialization and sub-specialization has occurred in orthopedic surgery similar to other fields of medicine. In 2016, an estimated 89.7% of orthopedic residency graduates elected to pursue subspecialization.[1] An area of special consideration due to its rapid growth is pediatric orthopedic surgery (POS).

The field of POS has changed tremendously over the past 2 decades. The interest in and number of fellowship positions has grown, and the climate of practice is ever evolving.[2] Due to the rapid growth of POS, many articles have been published examining the pediatric orthopedic workforce and how it is changing. Specifically, efforts have been made to quantify this growth and capture how the demographics of pediatric orthopedists are changing. As the number of surgeons trained annually has grown, concerns of market saturation and thus compensation have risen. The purpose of this review is to highlight these concepts and others to identify trends in recent literature allowing insight into potential areas of concern, and the future of this specialty.

GROWING INTEREST

The growth of POS can be attributed to many sources. Data from pediatric orthopedic fellowship match through San Francisco (SF) Match,[3] from its inception in 2010 to 2017, can provide quantifiable data showing growth in program numbers, available program spots, and number of applicants (**Fig. 1**). In this 8-year span, the number of fellowship programs grew from 36 to 47 (31% increase), allowing for a similar increase in the number of available positions (59%–75%; 27% increase). The number of applicants also rose during this time from 58 to 64 (10% increase), albeit to a lesser extent than the available positions. During this time, the match rate has increased by 8% (81% to 89%), presumably due to the slightly larger growth in

Disclosure: The authors have nothing to disclose.
[a] Department of Orthopaedic Surgery, Washington University in St. Louis, One Children's Place, 4S60, Suite 1B, St Louis, MO 63110, USA; [b] Pediatric and Adolescent Orthopedic Surgery, Washington University Orthopaedics, One Children's Place, 4S60, Suite 1B, St Louis, MO 63110, USA
* Corresponding author.
E-mail address: hosseinzadehp@wudosis.wustl.edu

MATCH DATA

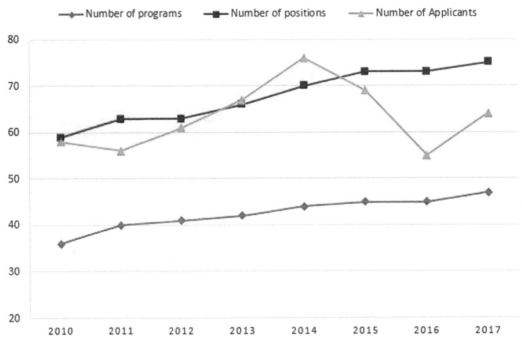

Fig. 1. Recent pediatric orthopedic fellowship data. (*Data from* SF Match Residency and Fellowship Matching Services. Pediatric Orthopaedic Fellowship. Residency and Fellowship Match. 2017. Available at: https://www.sfmatch.org/SpecialtyInsideAll.aspx?id=20&typ=1&name=Pediatric%2BOrthopaedic#. Accessed January 20, 2019.)

available positions compared with number of applicants.[3] These data do not tell the full story, however, as according to the Pediatric Orthopedic Society of North America (POSNA), from 2011 to 2014, 53 to 66 of open spots were filled by applicants who did not officially participate in the match.[4]

The 75 fellowship positions available in 2017 show tremendous growth when juxtaposed with only 30 open positions in the late 1990s.[5] Even more striking is that at the time only approximately a third of those spots were filled. The 10 pediatric orthopedists who were being trained to enter the workforce annually were overshadowed by 20 to 30 POSNA members who were retiring. A shortage was illuminated that needed to be addressed. According to Sawyer,[5] POSNA leadership and changing practice have helped combat attitudes that were creating this paradigm and create a shift to continued POS growth. As early as 2003, an increase in annual graduates was reported from the 10 per year in the late 1990s, to 39 per year in 2003, and up to 50 fellows in 2013.[6,7]

Further characterization of POS growth over the past 2 decades can be seen from increased POSNA membership. Between 1993 and 2014,

POSNA has seen a 59% increase in the number of active members: from 410 to 653. This increase can be attributed to a growth in the number of pediatric orthopedic fellows graduating from Accreditation Council for Graduate Medical Education–approved and non-approved programs each year, which itself increased from 39 to 50, between 2003 and 2013. In addition, POSNA candidate membership has also strikingly risen from 33 to 258 from 2000 to 2014.[7]

THE CHANGING WORKFORCE

Growth is often times accompanied by changing demographics of the original cohort and POS is no exception. Following suit with much of orthopedic surgery, the demographics of younger surgeons has greatly changed over the past few decades.[8,9] Specifically, the field of orthopedics has seen an increase in gender diversity. From 2010 to 2014, all subspecialties of orthopedic surgery saw an increase in female applicants, with POS reporting the largest proportion (25%), followed by foot and ankle (14%) and spine (3%). In terms of absolute numbers, POS comes second only to sports, with a total of 79 female applicants compared with 94. The large number of sports applicants could be attributed to the larger number of open positions. Moreover, it seems that the relative increase in the applicant pool is further supported by a higher overall fellowship match success rate for women compared with their male counterparts (96% vs 81%; $P<.001$).[10] This suggests that female applicants are desired in various fields of orthopedics; however, a subanalysis would be able to better shed light on which subspecialties specifically.

Although progress toward greater gender diversity in orthopedics has been made over the years, there is still great work to be done. More than half of medical school seats are occupied by women; however, fewer than 15% of orthopedic surgery residents are women.[10–12] Orthopedics has traditionally been a field with low representation by women and all trends suggest that this is slowly changing, with pediatric orthopedics leading the way.

Furthermore, POSNA membership has once again helped quantify some of these changes. For example, in 2014, 19% of active members and 34% of candidate members were women. This is in comparison with only 4.4% of members of the American Academy of Orthopedic Surgeons.[7,10] Sawyer and colleagues[7] reported that if this ratio was extrapolated to 2025, POSNA members would be 41% women.

In addition, approximately two-thirds of POSNA members are older than 50. Presumably, within the next 10 to 15 years, this group will approach the age of retirement.[7] With an increasing number of pediatric orthopedic surgeons training, and two-thirds of POSNA members retiring, the age distribution of POSNA members is anticipated to shift toward a younger demographic with increased female representation.

CASELOAD

The caseload of pediatric orthopedic surgeons demonstrates great variability depending on the setting of practice, namely private versus academic. A 2014 survey from the American Academy of Pediatrics (AAP) Section on Orthopedics (SOOr) surveyed 856 POSNA and 141 AAP-SOOr members to determine the distribution of practice settings. Their results are summarized in Table 1, with most pediatric orthopaedists choosing academic practice.[13] Practice locations and preferences have not changed substantially compared with the last AAP survey from 1998 as a part of the Future of Pediatric Education II (FOPE II) project.

Table 1
Results of Academy of Pediatrics Section on Orthopedics survey on workplace demographics

Work Demographics of Respondents	Percent of Respondents, %
Practice type	
Medical School/university	42
Specialty group	24
Multispecialty group	10
Pediatric group	7
Community hospital	5
Employment status	
Children's hospital	38
University employee	29
Private practice	25
Other	8
Military	1
Community type	
Urban, not inner city	46
Urban, inner city	31
Suburban	20
Rural	3

Adapted from Hosseinzadeh P, Copley L, Ruch-Ross H, et al. Current issues affecting the practice of pediatric orthopaedic surgeons: results of the 2014 Workforce Survey of American Academy of Pediatrics Section on Orthopaedics. J Pediatr Orthop 2018;38(1):e14–e19; with permission.

Amoli and colleagues[14] conducted a 2015 POSNA survey of new and well-established members investigating differences in attitudes and practice preferences between male and female pediatric orthopedists. Interestingly, they found recent female graduates were much more likely to choose academic practice than their male counterparts (72% vs 48%, $P<.001$). Moreover, female POSNA members reported a lower weekly operative case volume.[14]

The same survey outlined that most respondents receive referrals from general pediatricians (97%) and family medicine clinicians (92%), with most respondents reporting an increase in the last year of referrals (78%) and complexity of referrals (57%). This growth was perceived as sustained, as over the past 5 years, they also reported increased clinical volume (68%) and increased surgical volume (54%).[14]

With a growing number of pediatric orthopedic surgeons being trained annually, and perceived increased volume, Hosseinzadeh and colleagues[6] used the American Board of Ortho-pedic Surgeons (ABOS) Part II case log database to identify trends in case volume of pediatric or-thopedic surgeons in the first 2 years of practice between 2004 and 2014. The investigators looked at the relationship between number of applicants in POS and caseload over a 6-month case log, and found that although there was a consistent growth in the applicant pool during this period (15 in 2004, to 44 in 2014), the total case load also increased from 2142 to 4160. Importantly, this allowed the number of cases per applicant to stay stable over that period, showing a constant increase in supply with the growing demand.[4,6]

Further investigation done by Hosseinzadeh and colleagues[1] using the ABOS database from 2004 to 2014, was done to find what proportion of pediatric cases were being operated on by which specialty of orthopedists. The investiga-tors identified a total of 102,424 pediatric cases performed by candidates. As expected, there was a steady 65% decline in cases performed by adult surgeons, compared with a 168% in-crease in those done by pediatric orthopedic surgeons during that time (Fig. 2). Interestingly, when the patients were divided into non-adolescent (<13 years old) and adolescent (>13 years old), the increase in treatment by pe-diatric orthopedic surgeons was even more stag-gering (133% vs 244% increase) demonstrating where most of the case growth was coming from.[1] It appeared that the growth of cases was a shift, predominantly of adolescent cases, from adult surgeons, now being operated by pe-diatric orthopaedists.

Breakdown by specific procedure type: spine, sports, and trauma can be seen in Fig. 3. Pediatric sports medicine cases grew from only 7% of cases being performed by pe-diatric orthopedists in 2004, to 28% in 2014. Similarly, in terms of pediatric trauma, upper ex-tremity injuries grew from 12% to 43%, and lower extremity trauma from 12% to 47%. Although these show significant growth, these 3 areas convey that more than half of pediatric cases are still being treated by adult orthopedic surgeons. This is contrary to pediatric spine cases, in which the increase during the 11-year time span was from 54% in 2004 to 83% in 2014, leaving little room for future growth. These data were taken from surgeons in their first 2 years of practice, recording a 6-month case log. Importantly, the number of cases done per applicant stayed the same over this time span.[1]

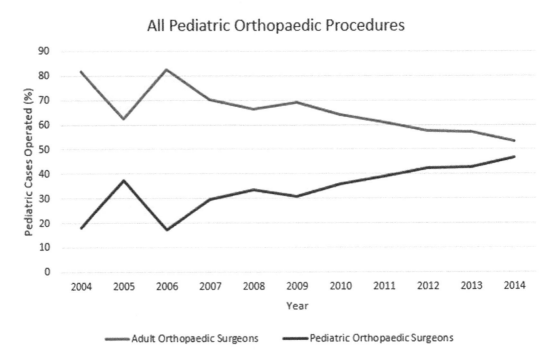

Fig. 2. Pediatric procedures operated on by adult versus pediatric surgeons using ABOS database, from 2004 to 2014. (*Adapted from* Hosseinzadeh P, Obey MR, Nielsen E, et al. Orthopaedic care for children: who provides it? How has it changed over the past decade? Analysis of the database of the American Board of Orthopaedic Surgery. J Pediatr Orthop 2019;39(3):e227–e231; with permission.)

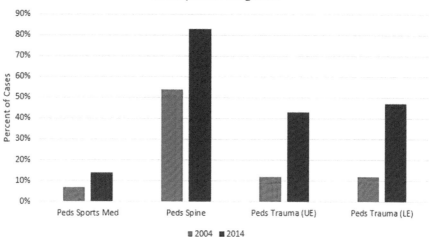

Fig. 3. Pediatric cases categorized by type of injury using ABOS database, from 2004 to 2014. LE, lower extremity; Peds, pediatrics; UE, upper extremity. (*Data from* Hosseinzadeh P, Obey MR, Nielsen E, et al. Orthopaedic Care for Children: Who Provides It? How Has It Changed Over the Past Decade? Analysis of the Database of the American Board of Orthopaedic Surgery. J Pediatr Orthop 2019;39(3):e227–e231.)

Although the proportion of pediatric cases operated on by adult orthopedic surgeons declined overall during this time, adult specialists in the realm of hand and upper extremity, sports medicine, and trauma specifically treated an increased number of pediatric cases during this period.[1] These may be areas of future growth for pediatric orthopedists, or areas of future subspecialization branching from pediatric orthopedics. Currently, areas of POS, such as foot and ankle, limb deformity, spine, and hip, have already become dominated by pediatric orthopedists treating more than 80% of the cases, perhaps hindering significant future growth.[1]

Overall, it seems that the pediatric caseload has been sufficient for most practicing pediatric orthopedists; 87% of recent fellowship-trained POS surveyed reported satisfaction with their current volume of pediatric cases. Those who are not satisfied with current volume attribute it to various issues, including competition from partners or other surgeons and actual volume deficiencies (**Fig. 4**).[4]

EXPANDING FIELDS

Four percent to 8% of orthopedic residents have recently gone on to pursue multiple fellowships.[15–17] Two recent studies identifying fellowship trends in the ABOS Part II candidate database found the most common combinations of such to be pediatrics and sports medicine.[2,18] During 2005 to 2015, 15% of pediatric orthopedic fellowship graduates pursued a dual fellowship, approximately half of which was in sports medicine. The percentage of pediatric orthopedic fellowship graduates completing another fellowship increased from just 5% between 2005 and 2008, to more than 28% in 2014 to 2015 ($P = .0001$), suggesting that this trend may actually be increasing.[2] This fellowship combination has become so common that there has been a dramatic rise in collaboration and efforts to organize specific pediatric sports medicine research groups (ie, ROCK [Research in Osteochondritis of the Knee], PRISM [Pediatric Research in Sports Medicine Society], PLUTO [Pediatric ACL: Understanding Treatment Outcomes], and FACTS [Function After Adolescent Clavicle Trauma and Surgery]).[15]

Obey and colleagues[15] looked at the ABOS Part II certification applicant case log over an 11-year period (2004–2014) to quantify who is performing pediatric sports medicine cases. They found that the percentage of sports medicine cases being treated by dual-fellowship–trained (pediatric and sports medicine fellowship) surgeons grew from 2.1% in 2004, to 21.4% in 2014. Furthermore, on a per-surgeon basis, the dual-fellowship–trained surgeons performed 5 times more cases than all other subspecialty candidates. With an increase in the number of surgeons pursuing

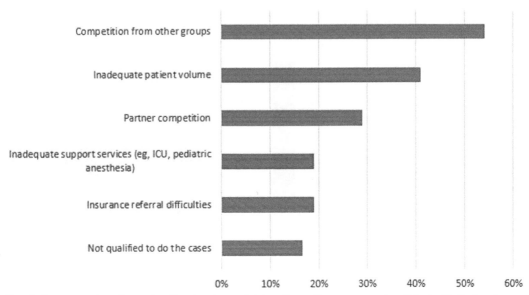

Fig. 4. Demonstration of perceived barriers by pediatric orthopedic surgeons not satisfied with their volume of pediatric cases. ICU, intensive care unit. (*Adapted from* Glotzbecker MP, Shore BJ, Fletcher ND, et al. Early career experience of pediatric orthopaedic fellows: what to expect and need for their services. J Pediatr Orthop 2016;36(4):429–432; with permission.)

dual-fellowship in these 2 fields, the investigators suggested that there may be the development of a new subspecialty.

Further evidence was seen in the 2016 POSNA survey of recent (2013–2014) pediatric orthopedic fellowship graduates; 30% of this group indicated completion of an additional fellowship.[4,6] This number is in line with the findings by Hosseinzadeh and colleagues,[2] confirming that the subspecialization in POS is increasing. It is difficult to ascertain the etiology of increasing subspecialization; however, increased market competition in academic centers and larger cities certainly plays a role and needs to be evaluated in future studies.

Areas of Future Growth

In addition to pediatric sports medicine as an emerging field, Hosseinzadeh and colleagues[1] shed light on specific areas of future growth in the realm of pediatric orthopedics. Specifically, pediatric trauma is currently an area without full pediatric orthopedic reach. Pediatric orthopedists treated only 53.4% of soft tissue injuries, 47.2% of lower extremity injuries, and 42.5% of upper extremity injuries between 2004 and 2014. Moreover, although specific treatment of traumatic pediatric injuries has risen in the past decade, the levels are still relatively low, with femur fractures (65%) and supracondylar humerus

fractures (61%) still being managed by many adult orthopedists.

Pediatric trauma, sports medicine, and hand and upper extremity offer great potential for future POS growth in the coming years. These areas have seen an increase in the absolute number of cases paired with relatively low current rates of treatment by pediatric orthopedists. With such a high proportion of cases being treated by non-pediatric orthopedists, there is an opportunity for a shift in management. The etiology of the rise in cases has not been clearly established for all fields. However, with regard to sports, there has been some suggestion that the increase may be due to some combination of a transition to single-sport specialization by young athletes or an increase in youth sports participation altogether.[19]

AREAS OF CONCERN

The pediatric orthopedic workforce has seen tremendous change over the years, and recent efforts, including a 2014 AAP-SOOr and a 2016 POSNA survey, have been made to capture the opinions of its members.

Competition

POS in the past has been perceived as a major undersupplied subspecialty of orthopedics; however, recent surveys convey that this attitude is changing.[13,20] Nearly a third (28%) of pediatric orthopedic surgeons who responded to the POSNA survey believe that too many pediatric orthopedists are being trained, whereas more than 75% of AAP-SOOr member respondents reported increased geographic competition, with most (90%) indicating this competition was with other pediatric orthopedic subspecialists.[4,13]

With population growth amounting to only approximately 1% to 2% per year in the United States, and many pediatric conditions having a fixed incidence (clubfoot, developmental dysplasia of the hip, and scoliosis), it is understandable how increased training of pediatric orthopedists can be worrisome.[7] Currently, it is estimated that 20% of new job offers for recent fellowship-trained pediatric orthopedic surgeons come from replacement of a retiring senior partner.[4] Potentially, this would mean 80% of new jobs should be coming from sources such as growth of an established practice or creation of a new one.

In addition to increased saturation of pediatric orthopedists in some markets, another source of competition has come from nonsurgical providers. The increase in nurse practitioners, nonoperative orthopedic surgeons, and physician assistants is hard to quantify. The Pediatric Orthopedic Practitioner Society has provided some assessment in this change. Their membership has grown from 47 members in 2000, to 130 members in 2014.[7] Although other providers increase competition, the AAP-SOOr survey revealed that more than half of respondents planned to hire a nonphysician provider due to increased volume of referrals.[13]

Furthermore, other surgical specialties have associated surgeon:population ratio benchmarks, whereas none has been established for POS.[7] These benchmarks provide valuable insight into quantification of geographic market saturation. The lack of such benchmarks in POS may be due to the growth in this field. POS is still rapidly growing, with a large contribution of caseload growth coming from a shift in pediatric surgical cases from adult orthopedists.[1] Inevitably, this shift in operative treatment will reach a steady state allowing surgeon:population ratio benchmarks to be developed for pediatric orthopedics.

Results of the AAP-SOOr survey revealed that 28% of respondents planned on retiring or limiting their practice within the next few years. The most common of these reasons seemed to be physical wear, family needs, and emotional stress.[13] This number will most likely increase as more than two-thirds of POSNA members are 50 years or older (mean; 52), and thus more and more members will reach the age of retirement within the next 10 to 15 years.[7]

Compensation

Undoubtedly, reimbursement plays a major role in residency as well as fellowship choice for many applicants. A 2007 survey from American Orthopedic Association demonstrated that 59% of those who completed the survey believed that POS was the most underrepresented subspecialty. Contributing factors were attributed to perceived lower reimbursement, volume of cases, and malpractice liability.[7]

Sawyer and colleagues[7] used the compensation data from The Medical Group Management Association (MGMA) in 2014 (Fig. 5) to show relative growth in POS salaries from 2006. MGMA data include 60,000 providers in 170 different specialties to compile these data. When looking at percent change in salary among pediatric general surgeons, general orthopedic surgeons, pediatricians, and pediatric orthopedic surgeons, during that time frame, POS showed the smallest increase (21%). The largest growth was noted to be pediatric general surgeons (46%), followed by pediatricians (26%) and general orthopedic surgeons (33%).

In a 2016 survey demonstrating salary attitudes among recent fellowship-trained pediatric orthopedic surgeons, Glotzbecker and colleagues[4] reported the following: 44% think their salary is "just right," 36.5% believe their salary is "too low but is expected to increase to an appropriate level," and 12.5% believe their salary is too low and will not increase.

Although compensation and competition are areas of concern for some, the same 2016, 36-question, survey found that 91% of respondents were very or extremely satisfied with their fellowship experience and 97.5% received at least 1 job offer on fellowship completion.[4]

Other Concerns

The AAP-SOOr survey noted other areas of concern as well. Overall, electronic medical records were seen as hindering productivity. Common reasons for this negative outlook were inability to see as many patients (63%) and a hindrance to physician-patient relationships (43%).[13]

Although variable, the best estimate of hours per week that pediatric orthopedic surgeons work is nearly 60 hours per week. This figure has not changed much from its 1998

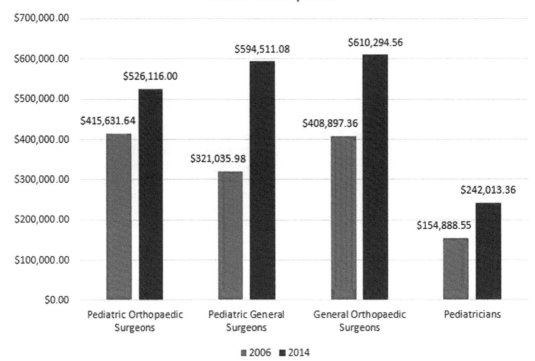

Fig. 5. MGMA data showing pediatric orthopedic salary information. (*Data from* Sawyer JR, Jones KC, Copley LA, et al. Pediatric Orthopaedic Workforce in 2014: Current Workforce and Projections for the Future. J Pediatr Orthop 2017;37(1):59–66.)

estimate of 64 hours.[13] Understandably, work hours may be a concern from some; however, 60 hours appears to be much lower than other subspecialties of orthopedics and did not appear to be a concern for the surveyed surgeons.

Trauma care has been in the limelight of concerns as well. A 2015 POSNA Membership survey demonstrated that although 83% of pediatric orthopedists consider trauma call an integral part of their practice, only 53% are satisfied with the experience. Common issues include only 47% having access to a designated trauma operating room (OR) and only 43% of pediatric orthopedists reporting a stipend for taking call. As expected, younger age, financial compensation, and available support increase perceived satisfaction. Trends appear to be headed in the right direction, as trauma OR access has increased 196% and proportion of surgeons receiving call compensation has also increased 154% since 2006.[21] However, half of pediatric orthopedists are still not satisfied with their call experience, and further studies need to investigate how to alleviate this level of dissatisfaction.

THE FUTURE OF PEDIATRIC ORTHOPEDIC SURGERY

Pediatric orthopedics is a growing, healthy, and dynamic field, but not without its challenges. To continue on this upward trajectory in a balanced way, the subspecialty must look to the future. Consistent efforts should be made to closely and meticulously monitor the pediatric orthopedic workforce to predict future need, quickly address obstacles, and improve practice efficiencies. The field should continue to work toward increasing interest in the field by focusing on medical student and resident education.

Predicting Future Need

Predicting the exact future need for pediatric orthopedic surgeons may be impossible due to the complex relationship among economic, government, insurance/health care system, and training factors. In addition, there is also an increasing demand for referrals to trauma or teaching hospitals for management of traumatic pediatric injuries,[22,23] as well as demand from local communities for pediatric specialists and subspecialists for treatment of their children's injuries/complaints.[24] This does not mean that strong efforts should not be made to closely approximate the need and attempt to match supply with demand. Sawyer and colleagues[7] searched the POSNA, SF Match, Kids' Inpatient Database (KID), MGMA ,and US Census data and identified several trends to expect in the coming years:

- The supply of pediatric orthopedic surgeons and physician extenders has increased significantly. The number of female POSNA members has increased significantly.
- A significant number of experienced of pediatric orthopedic surgeons will be leaving the workforce in the next 10 to 15 years, which may balance out the increased supply.
- Gross domestic product and population growth, which drive the demand for health care services are expected to remain stable in the short-term.
- The scope of practice of pediatric orthopedic surgeons has expanded significantly into the sports, hand, and spine surgery fields.

As recommended by Sawyer and colleagues,[7] continued reassessment of the need for pediatric orthopedic surgeons should be performed regularly and changes can be made accordingly.

Multidisciplinary Approach and Practice

Physician extenders employed by surgeons, such as physician assistants and nurse practitioners, can be used to build an efficient and lucrative practice. This practice model makes additional sense when considering that nonoperative management of pediatric orthopedic problems comprises approximately 50% of pediatric orthopedic surgeon income.[19,20] As the scope of practice of physician extenders expands, there is a natural point of contention that may arise in which certain pediatric problems should be more appropriately treated by physicians rather than physician extenders. Patient care may suffer if, for example, in a cost-cutting measure, physician extenders are allowed to practice more independently without some level of physician oversight for complex problems. Clinical research in this sphere is important and much needed.

The scarcity of training in musculoskeletal medicine in medical school carries over to a lack of comfort in managing orthopedic issues by nonorthopedic physicians in residency and practice.[25–27] Pediatric, family, and internal medicine training programs should consider including more musculoskeletal education into their curriculums. Collaboration with orthopedic, rheumatology, and radiology departments would go a long way toward closing the knowledge gap in musculoskeletal medicine. Efforts have been put forth by the AAP and POSNA for continuing musculoskeletal education for primary care providers.[24]

Education and Mentorship

Early exposure to a field in medical school through coursework, hands-on clinical experience, and mentorship are often cited as the most important factors in career choice. Orthopedics, however, is quite unique as a field in that a disproportionately large number of residency applicants choose to go into the field before, or very early on in medical school.[28] Although both orthopedic-bound and non–orthopedic-bound medical students are most significantly affected by third-year and fourth-year rotations, orthopedic-bound students are more likely to be impacted by experiences and people before medical school than non–orthopedic-bound applicants. They are also less likely to report a specific faculty member as the most important person influencing their career choice. Orthopedic surgery is clearly very self-selecting, and the lack of exposure in the medical school curriculum deserves criticism.

This is compounded by the underrepresentation of musculoskeletal medicine in US medical schools, which needs to be addressed expeditiously.[25–27] In 2006, our institution created a required 1-month musculoskeletal surgery (orthopedic surgery, plastic surgery, or neurosurgical spine) experience within the traditional 3-month surgery clerkship.[29] Students are paired with assigned faculty for two 2-week blocks and also participate in twice-weekly lectures by faculty and senior residents, weekly physical examination sessions, and 3 or 4 nights of adult trauma or pediatric call. Medical students get to work closely with residents, who nationally have been found to provide 20% to 70% of the clinical teaching for medical students, and get the opportunity to build new mentorship connections with people who have a more up-to-date understanding of being a medical student than senior faculty mentors.[30] Since the change, our institution has noted an 81% relative increase (17% to 30%) of female applicants to orthopedic surgery. Before the curriculum change, our institution female applicant rate was on par with the national average of approximately 15%. Similar changes were noted for underrepresented minority applicants, with a relative increase of 101% (10% to 21%). Through this experience, medical students are also able to more easily identify faculty mentors, which is very important, especially for those who did not consider orthopedics before medical school.

After an exposure to orthopedics, medical students could be encouraged to pursue a pediatric orthopedic focus through their clinical rotations and research. Multiple scholarships are available through the International Pediatric Orthopedic Symposium, the AAP-SOOr, and POSNA in support of pediatric orthopedic research and mentorship. The efforts described also could be applicable to resident education and recruitment toward pediatric orthopedics.

SUMMARY

All in all, the field of POS has changed in many ways over the past 2 decades. It has changed in terms of growth and interest, demographics, and opinions of members. Periodic survey of the workforce allows leadership in the field to continue to promote healthy growth, patient safety, as well as address concerns as they arise. The surveys of members and the literature on POS confirm that there has been a sustained balance of interest and opportunity in growth of applicant numbers as well as fellowship spots.[8] Moreover, pediatric orthopedics has been leading the way in diversity in the realm of orthopedics with respect to gender, and it seems as though this trend will continue into the foreseeable future.[11,14] Concerns of competition are valid and appear to be rising; however, case load data suggest that with increased training of pediatric orthopedists, there seems to be adequate increase in cases.[18] Periodic workforce analysis should continue to gauge any changes in attitudes or workload.

REFERENCES

1. Hosseinzadeh P, Obey MR, Nielsen E, et al. Orthopaedic care for children: who provides it? How has it changed over the past decade? Analysis of the database of the American Board of Orthopaedic Surgery. J Pediatr Orthop 2018;39(3):e227–31.

2. Hosseinzadeh P, Louer C, Sawyer J, et al. Subspecialty training among graduates of pediatric orthopaedic fellowships: an 11-year analysis of the database of American Board of Orthopaedic Surgery. J Pediatr Orthop 2018;38(5):293–6.

3. SF Match: residency and fellowship matching services. Pediatric Orthopaedic Fellowship. Residency and fellowship match. 2017. Available at: https://www.sfmatch.org/SpecialtyInsideAll.aspx?id=20&typ=1&name=Pediatric%2BOrthopaedic#. Accessed January 20, 2019.

4. Glotzbecker MP, Shore BJ, Fletcher ND, et al. Early career experience of pediatric orthopaedic fellows: what to expect and need for their services. J Pediatr Orthop 2016;36(4):429–32.

5. Sawyer JR. The changing face of pediatric orthopedics. Am J Orthop (Belle Mead NJ) 2016;45(1):10–1.

6. Hosseinzadeh P, DeVries CA, Nielsen E, et al. Changes in the practice of pediatric orthopaedic surgeons over the past decade: analysis of the database of the American Board of Orthopaedic Surgery. J Pediatr Orthop 2018;38(8):e486–9.

7. Sawyer JR, Jones KC, Copley LA, et al. Pediatric orthopaedic workforce in 2014: current workforce and projections for the future. J Pediatr Orthop 2017;37(1):59–66.

8. Daniels EW, French K, Murphy LA, et al. Has diversity increased in orthopaedic residency programs since 1995? Clin Orthop Relat Res 2012;470(8):2319–24.

9. Van Heest AE, Fishman F, Agel J. A 5-year update on the uneven distribution of women in orthopaedic surgery residency training programs in the United States. J Bone Joint Surg Am 2016;98(15):e64.

10. Cannada LK. Women in orthopaedic fellowships: what is their match rate, and what specialties do they choose? Clin Orthop Relat Res 2016;474(9):1957–61.

11. Huntington WP, Haines N, Patt JC. What factors influence applicants' rankings of orthopaedic surgery residency programs in the National Resident Matching Program? Clin Orthop Relat Res 2014;472(9):2859–66.

12. Van Heest AE, Agel J. The uneven distribution of women in orthopaedic surgery resident training programs in the United States. J Bone Joint Surg Am 2012;94(2):e9.

13. Hosseinzadeh P, Copley L, Ruch-Ross H, et al. Current issues affecting the practice of pediatric orthopaedic surgeons: results of the 2014 workforce survey of American Academy of Pediatrics Section on Orthopaedics. J Pediatr Orthop 2018;38(1):e14–9.

14. Amoli MA, Flynn JM, Edmonds EW, et al. Gender differences in pediatric orthopaedics: what are the implications for the future workforce? Clin Orthop Relat Res 2016;474(9):1973–8.

15. Obey MR, Lamplot J, Nielsen ED, et al. Pediatric sports medicine, a new subspeciality in orthopedics: an analysis of the surgical volume of candidates for the American Board of Orthopaedic Surgery Part II Certification Exam over the past decade. J Pediatr Orthop 2019;39(1):e71–6.

16. Horst PK, Choo K, Bharucha N, et al. Graduates of orthopaedic residency training are increasingly

subspecialized: a review of the American Board of Orthopaedic Surgery Part II database. J Bone Joint Surg Am 2015;97(10):869–75.

17. Hariri S, York SC, O'Connor MI, et al. Career plans of current orthopaedic residents with a focus on sex-based and generational differences. J Bone Joint Surg Am 2011;93(5):e16.

18. DePasse JM, Daniels AH, Durand W, et al. Completion of multiple fellowships by orthopedic surgeons: analysis of the American Board of Orthopaedic Surgery Certification Database. Orthopedics 2018;41(1):e33–7.

19. Smucny M, Parikh SN, Pandya NK. Consequences of single sport specialization in the pediatric and adolescent athlete. Orthop Clin North Am 2015; 46(2):249–58.

20. Salsberg ES, Grover A, Simon MA, et al. An AOA critical issue. Future physician workforce requirements: implications for orthopaedic surgery education. J Bone Joint Surg Am 2008;90(5): 1143–59.

21. Lind A, Latz K, Sinclair MR, et al. Pediatric orthopaedic surgeons dissatisfied in on-call practices despite improving call conditions. The 2015 POSNA membership survey regarding trauma care. J Pediatr Orthop 2018;38(2):e33–7.

22. Holt JB, Glass NA, Bedard NA, et al. Emerging U.S. national trends in the treatment of pediatric supracondylar humeral fractures. J Bone Joint Surg Am 2017;99(8):681–7.

23. Kasser JR. Location of treatment of supracondylar fractures of the humerus in children. Clin Orthop Relat Res 2005;434:110–3.

24. Schwend RM. The pediatric orthopaedics workforce demands, needs, and resources. J Pediatr Orthop 2009;29(7):653–60.

25. Friedman MH, Connell KJ, Olthoff AJ, et al. Medical student errors in making a diagnosis. Acad Med 1998;73(10 Suppl):S19–21.

26. Matzkin E, Smith EL, Freccero D, et al. Adequacy of education in musculoskeletal medicine. J Bone Joint Surg Am 2005;87(2):310–4.

27. DiGiovanni BF, Sundem LT, Southgate RD, et al. Musculoskeletal medicine is underrepresented in the American medical school clinical curriculum. Clin Orthop Relat Res 2016;474(4): 901–7.

28. Johnson AL, Sharma J, Chinchilli VM, et al. Why do medical students choose orthopaedics as a career? J Bone Joint Surg Am 2012;94(11):e78.

29. London DA, Calfee RP, Boyer MI. Impact of a musculoskeletal clerkship on orthopedic surgery applicant diversity. Am J Orthop (Belle Mead NJ) 2016;45(6):E347–51.

30. Wilson FC. Teaching by residents. Clin Orthop Relat Res 2007;454:247–50.

The Canary in the Coal Mine

Wellness Among Pediatric Orthopedic Surgeons

Rachel Y. Goldstein, MD, MPH[a],*, Jennifer M. Weiss, MD[b]

KEYWORDS

- Physician wellness • Mindfulness • Burnout • Pediatric orthopedics

KEY POINTS

- Occupational burnout is a pervasive problem in pediatric orthopedics.
- Mindfulness is a potential antidote to burnout.
- Systemic changes are required to combat burnout.

WELLNESS AS IT PERTAINS TO THE PEDIATRIC ORTHOPEDIST

The anecdotal perception of the pediatric orthopedic profession is one of pride and purpose. After all, treating children with musculoskeletal injuries and pathology is a high calling achieved only after years of training and continuously proving oneself clinically, academically, and personally. A study of American orthopedic surgeons over the age of 50 showed that 80% demonstrated high job satisfaction.[1] Larger cross-sectional studies report that approximately one-half of American orthopedic surgeons are satisfied with their work–life balance and have high job satisfaction.[2,3] A 2009 systemic review of 97 American jobs found that factors associated with physician satisfaction include both physician factors (age and specialty), and job factors (job demands, job control, collegial support, income, and incentives).[4]

As physician and clinician wellness has come to be a pervasive conversation in the medical field, it does not seem that there are any fields that are immune to burnout, which is an enemy of wellness. Occupational burnout consists of 3 key elements: emotional exhaustion, depersonalization, and a perceived lack of personal accomplishments.[5] A survey of almost 7000 physicians conducted by the American Medical Association compared the prevalence of burnout and physicians' satisfaction with work–life balance with the general US population relative to 2011 and 2014.[6] They found that the percentage of US physicians who met criteria for burnout increased from 45.0% in 2011 to 54.5% in 2014. Specifically, the burnout rate for orthopedic surgeons increased from 48.3% to 59.6%.

In 2018, the Pediatric Orthopedic Society of North America (POSNA) called for a task force to be created to investigate physician wellness in the pediatric orthopedic community. The task force identified their first order of business to define the scope of the problem. The POSNA membership was surveyed and 47% responded. The results of the survey confirmed that the problem of burnout is real and prevalent. More than one-third of the respondents identified themselves as burned out. The survey found that 3.5% of respondents felt "completely burned out and often wonder if I can go on. I am at the point where I may need some changes or may need to seek some sort of help," 7.3% felt that "the symptoms of burnout that I'm experiencing won't go away. I think about frustration at work a lot." In addition, 26.9% agreed

Disclosure Statement: The authors have nothing to disclose.
a Pediatric Orthopaedics, Children's Hospital Los Angeles, 4650 Sunset Boulevard MS 69, Los Angeles, CA 90027, USA; b Permanente Medical Group, 4760 Sunset Boulevard, Los Angeles, CA 90027, USA
* Corresponding author.
E-mail address: rgoldstein@chla.usc.edu

0030-5898/19/© 2019 Elsevier Inc. All rights reserved.

that "I am definitely burning out and have one or more symptoms of burnout, such as physical and emotional exhaustion" (Table 1). The problem is real, and even pediatric orthopedists are clearly affected by the burnout epidemic.

The rate of suicide is known to be higher among physicians compared with the general population[7] and self-reported rates of depression among physicians range from 11% to 46%.[8–11] Mental impairment is known to be a devastating problem among physicians in general, with orthopedic surgeons proving to be no exception. It is estimated that we lose 400 physicians to suicide every year.[12] Pamela Wible delivered a poignant keynote address to the 19th Annual Chicago Orthopedic Symposium, entitled "33 Orthopedic Surgeon Suicides, How to Prevent #34." The presentation has circulated on social media, educating thousands of people about those we have lost. To prevent the next, engagement and transparency with the problem must amplify.

Burnout is a close cousin to depression. The symptoms of burnout decrease quality of life. Emotional exhaustion is associated with physical exhaustion and poor judgment, depersonalization results in cynicism and impaired relationships with patients and colleagues, and feelings of low personal achievement lead to decreased effectiveness and productivity.[13,14] In addition, physician burnout increases the rate of medical errors. Shanafelt and associates[15] found that, for each point increase in a depersonalization score, there was an 11% increase in the risk of

a medical error and for each point increase in emotional exhaustion there was a 5% risk of a medical error. Patients report decreased satisfaction when their doctors and team are burned out.[16] Last, there is an increased rate of medical lawsuits associated with disengaged doctors.[17] After all, as Theodore Roosevelt said, "nobody cares how much you know until they know how much you care"

A unique consideration is necessary for women surgeons and their risk of burnout. POSNA has the highest percentage of women among orthopedic societies. As of 2016, 18% of active POSNA members were women, and this proportion is expected to increase to 40% by 2025.[18] As such, POSNA is the natural leader to support women surgeons in their different challenges. The POSNA survey found that women surgeons were more likely to report burnout than male surgeons. This higher level of burnout may be linked to the higher likelihood of workplace bullying and harassment toward women. A 2018 survey conducted by the American Academy of Orthopedic Surgeons and reported in American Academy of Orthopedic Surgeons Now December 2018 found that discrimination was reported at a much higher rate in females (84%) than in males (59%). Females also reported higher rates of bullying, harassment, and sexual harassment. Other theories may include pay disparity; implicit bias received from doctors, clinicians, and patients; and balancing pregnancy and childbearing during training or practice.

To date, there has been a greater emphasis on the surgeon themselves to strengthen and become more resilient. It is imperative to change focus to the health care system itself, as well as the hospital and environment in which surgeons practice. The canary's job in the coal mine is to sing, and when the coal mine becomes too toxic for the canary to sing, this is a harbinger for the coal miners. This analogy can be applied to our current state of physician well-being. The surgeon canaries are strong and resilient, but when the coal mine system becomes too toxic for pediatric orthopedic surgeons to "sing," it is time to change the coal mine rather than further strengthen the surgeon canaries.

The role of POSNA has taken on 2 aspects: individual well-being efforts and institutional culture changes. Well-being efforts continue to be important as we bring up young and aspiring surgeons and remind our midcareer and senior surgeons to eat well, sleep enough, exercise, and perhaps practice mindfulness and gratitude. Normalizing and promoting self-care is a culture

Table 1 Results from the survey of POSNA members	
"I enjoy my work. I have no symptoms of burnout."	15.38%
"Occasionally I am under stress, and I don't always have as much energy as I once did, but I don't feel burned out."	46.85%
"I am definitely burning out and have one or more symptoms of burnout, such as physical and emotional exhaustion."	26.92%
"The symptoms of burnout that I'm experiencing won't go away. I think about frustration at work a lot."	7.34%
"I feel completely burned out and often wonder if I can go on. I am at the point where I may need some changes or may need to seek some sort of help."	3.50%

shift, and modeling and promoting these behaviors from the leadership of the field is imperative.

However, healthy habits require time and space. The second role of POSNA is to equip our membership to be agents of culture change within their own practice settings and home institutions. Barriers to wellness and ignitors of burnout and depression include high call volume, lack of access to operating rooms during daylight hours, increased patient volume, decreased help in the office and hospital settings, and electronic medical record responsibilities. Cost drives many of these barriers. In contrast, the financial and emotional costs of losing a physician or clinician to burnout and depression temporarily or permanently is large, and has not received sufficient study.

Burnout is an occupational hazard for pediatric orthopedists and their teams, and is characterized by exhaustion of physical or emotional strength as a result of prolonged stress or frustration. A low level of perceived personal accomplishment accompanies this state, and 20% to 60% of physicians report burnout. Burnout correlates with a higher rate of medical malpractice and medical errors.[19,20] Medical leaders and bosses are not immune to burnout, as Shanafelt and colleagues[21] showed us that most ear, nose, and throat and obstetrics and gynecology chairs reported moderate burnout. "Those surgeons most dedicated to their profession and their patient may very well be most susceptible to burnout."[22]

Mindfulness is a well-studied antidote to burnout. Although mindfulness and other canary-strengthening strategies cannot replace strategies to alleviate toxicity in the coal mine, the benefits of mindfulness are outstanding. "Mindfulness is awareness that arises through paying attention, on purpose, in the present moment, non-judgementally," says Kabat-Zinn. "It's about knowing what is on your mind." In 2015, Dr Kahn wrote a striking piece in the New England Journal of Medicine entitled, "On Taking Notice—Learning Mindfulness from (Boston) Brahmins."[23] Dr Kahn suggests that "caring for the present moment, or allowing ourselves to be more mindful, is underrated as a technique for both improving care and increasing professional satisfaction."

A 2013 pilot study examined the effects of an 18-hour mindfulness course followed by 10 to 20 minutes per day of practice among primary care clinicians.[24] The work involved sitting, movement, speaking, listening, compassion for self and others, and application to medical practice and everyday life. They reported decreased burnout, decreased depression, decreased anxiety, decreased stress, and increased resilience among those studied. "A Multicenter Study of Physician Mindfulness and Health Care Quality" published in the Annals of Family Medicine showed that the practice of mindfulness correlated with patients feeling better heard, reporting better experiences, and rating their doctors higher.[25] A study examining a short course of mindfulness practice among 38 nurses found decreased stress after 1 month that was maintained 1 month later. A 5-minute mindfulness meditation before a shift for nurses in a pediatric intensive care unit correlated with improvements in the Nursing Stress Scale, the Maslach Burnout Inventory, the Mindfulness Attention Awareness scale, and the Self-Compassion Scale.[26]

The basics of the practice of mindfulness are presented in **Box 1**.

Opportunities for mindful practice in the day of a pediatric orthopedic surgeon include pauses that already happen in the day of a busy surgeon, such as during a scrub for the operating room, waiting for the sterile prep to dry, and waiting for patients to be roomed. Involving the team of nurses, technicians, other physicians, students, and trainees can amplify the benefits. As work is done with the hospitals and health care environment to decrease toxicity, we can and should focus on the resilience and health of the canary surgeon.

In conclusion, we are entering uncharted territory. Future directions for our work in the pediatric orthopedic community include an emphasis on the "coal mine." Future goals are to arm our membership with research and recommendations regarding advocating for systems that are designed for our doctors to provide the best care. We know that burnout is a risk when a surgeon cannot give a patient what she knows the patient needs. So systems-based interventions are the future in terms of physician wellness.

Box 1
Practice of mindfulness

When is the last time you sat silently for 90 seconds?

What if you sat silently for 90 seconds and rested your attention on your breathing?

What if you sat silently for 90 seconds, rested your attention on your breathing, AND noticed when your mind was wandering, and returned your attention back to the breathing?

Some topics that require research are implications of call ratio, scribes and advanced practitioner assistance, and trauma room access and their correlation to burnout and wellness.

REFERENCES

1. Farley FA, Kramer J, Watkins-Castillo S. Work satisfaction and retirement plans of orthopaedic surgeons 50 years of age and older. Clin Orthop Relat Res 2008;466(1):231–8.
2. Leigh JP, Kravitz RL, Schembri M, et al. Physician career satisfaction across specialties. Arch Intern Med 2002;162(14):1577–84.
3. Shanafelt TD, Boone S, Tan L, et al. Burnout and satisfaction with work-life balance among US physicians relative to the general US population. Arch Intern Med 2012;172(18):1377–85.
4. Scheurer D, McKean S, Miller J, et al. U.S. physician satisfaction: a systematic review. J Hosp Med 2009; 4(9):560–8.
5. Maslach C, Schaufeli WB, Leiter MP. Job burnout. Annu Rev Psychol 2001;52:397–422.
6. Shanafelt TD, Hasan O, Dyrbye LN, et al. Changes in burnout and satisfaction with work-life balance in physicians and the general US working population between 2011 and 2014. Mayo Clin Proc 2015; 90(12):1600–13.
7. Schernhammer ES, Colditz GA. Suicide rates among physicians: a quantitative and gender assessment (meta-analysis). Am J Psychiatry 2004; 161(12):2295–302.
8. Adams EF, Lee AJ, Pritchard CW, et al. What stops us from healing the healers: a survey of help-seeking behaviour, stigmatisation and depression within the medical profession. Int J Soc Psychiatry 2010;56(4):359–70.
9. Frank E, Dingle AD. Self-reported depression and suicide attempts among U.S. women physicians. Am J Psychiatry 1999;156(12):1887–94.
10. Hassan TM, Ahmed SO, White AC, et al. A postal survey of doctors' attitudes to becoming mentally ill. Clin Med (Lond) 2009;9(4):327–32.
11. Schwenk TL, Gorenflo DW, Leja LM. A survey on the impact of being depressed on the professional status and mental health care of physicians. J Clin Psychiatry 2008;69(4):617–20.
12. Gold KJ, Sen A, Schwenk TL. Details on suicide among US physicians: data from the National Violent Death Reporting System. Gen Hosp Psychiatry 2013;35(1):45–9.
13. Arora M, Diwan AD, Harris IA. Burnout in orthopaedic surgeons: a review. ANZ J Surg 2013;83(7–8): 512–5.
14. Daniels AH, DePasse JM, Kamal RN. Orthopaedic surgeon burnout: diagnosis, treatment, and prevention. J Am Acad Orthop Surg 2016;24(4):213–9.
15. Shanafelt TD, Balch CM, Bechamps G, et al. Burnout and medical errors among American surgeons. Ann Surg 2010;251(6):995–1000.
16. Shanafelt TD, Bradley KA, Wipf JE, et al. Burnout and self-reported patient care in an internal medicine residency program. Ann Intern Med 2002; 136(5):358–67.
17. Balch CM, Oreskovich MR, Dyrbye LN, et al. Personal consequences of malpractice lawsuits on American surgeons. J Am Coll Surg 2011;213(5): 657–67.
18. Amoli MA, Flynn JM, Edmonds EW, et al. Gender differences in pediatric orthopaedics: what are the implications for the future workforce? Clin Orthop Relat Res 2016;474(9):1973–8.
19. Chen KY, Yang CM, Lien CH, et al. Burnout, job satisfaction, and medical malpractice among physicians. Int J Med Sci 2013;10(11):1471–8.
20. Romani M, Ashkar K. Burnout among physicians. Libyan J Med 2014;9:23556.
21. Shanafelt TD, Gorringe G, Menaker R, et al. Impact of organizational leadership on physician burnout and satisfaction. Mayo Clin Proc 2015;90(4):432–40.
22. Balch CM, Shanafelt T. Combating stress and burnout in surgical practice: a review. Adv Surg 2010;44:29–47.
23. Kahn MW. On taking notice–learning mindfulness from (Boston) Brahmins. N Engl J Med 2015; 372(10):901–3.
24. Fortney L, Luchterhand C, Zakletskaia L, et al. Abbreviated mindfulness intervention for job satisfaction, quality of life, and compassion in primary care clinicians: a pilot study. Ann Fam Med 2013; 11(5):412–20.
25. Beach MC, Roter D, Korthuis PT, et al. A multicenter study of physician mindfulness and health care quality. Ann Fam Med 2013;11(5): 421–8.
26. Gauthier T, Meyer RM, Grefe D, et al. An on-the-job mindfulness-based intervention for pediatric ICU nurses: a pilot. J Pediatr Nurs 2015;30(2):402–9.

A Five-year Review of the Designated Leadership Positions of Pediatric Orthopaedic Society of North America: Where Do Women Stand?

Selina Poon, MD[a],*, Joshua Abzug, MD[b],
Michelle Caird, MD[c], Robert H. Cho, MD[a],
Marilan Luong, MPH[d], Jennifer M. Weiss, MD[e]

KEYWORDS

• Orthopedic • Women • Leadership • POSNA • Committees

KEY POINTS

• Female Pediatric Orthopaedic Society of North America (POSNA) members apply to committee positions and volunteer at a greater proportion than do their male counterparts.
• The increased gender diversity of the POSNA membership is not yet reflected in its current leadership hierarchy.
• Additional time is necessary to observe whether increased volunteerism by women in POSNA will translate into leadership roles in society.

BACKGROUND

The percentage of female orthopedic surgeons in the United States in 2016 was 6.6%, the lowest of all areas of medicine,[1] including other surgical subspecialties.[2–4] Despite near equal representation of women compared to men in medical schools since 2008, at 47% to 48%,[5] the percentage of women in orthopaedic surgery residency has ranged from 12% to 14% during that same time period.[6] Lack of exposure, negative perceptions about lifestyle, lack of diversity, lack of role models, misconceptions about the models the physical demands, and incompatibility with family life have all been suggested as explanations as to why women do not choose orthopedic surgery as a subspecialty.[4,7–9]

Within the subspecialties of orthopedic surgery, pediatric orthopedic fellowships enrolled a significantly greater percentage (29.52%) of female fellows than did all other orthopedic subspecialties, except oncology, from 2005 to 2015.[10] The Pediatric Orthopaedic Society of North America (POSNA) is one of the largest not-for-profit professional organizations within pediatric orthopedic surgery. There are more than 1400 members, including surgeons, non-surgeon physicians, and allied health professionals, whose practice is focused on pediatric

---

Disclosure Statement: Dr Robert H. Cho reports personal fees from DePuy Synthes Spine, personal fees from NuVasive, and personal fees from Ergobaby, outside the submitted work.
[a] Orthopaedic Surgery Department, Shriners for Children Medical Center, 909 South Fair Oaks Avenue, Pasadena, CA 91105, USA; [b] Department of Orthopaedics and Pediatrics, University of Maryland School of Medicine, 1 Texas Station Court, Suite 300, Timonium, MD 21093, USA; [c] Pediatric Orthopaedic Department, University of Michigan, 1540 East Hospital Drive, Ann Arbor, MI 48109, USA; [d] Research Department, Shriners for Children Medical Center, 909 South Fair Oaks Avenue, Pasadena, CA 91105, USA; [e] Pediatric Orthopaedic Department, Kaiser Permanente, 4760 Sunset Boulevard, Los Angeles, CA 90027, USA
* Corresponding author.
E-mail address: spoon@shrinenet.org

orthopedics. The distribution between men and women within POSNA surpasses both the national average in orthopedic surgery and 15 of the 19 American Academy of Orthopaedic Surgeons Board of Specialty Societies member organizations.[11,12] The reasons behind the success of pediatric orthopedics in attracting women is unknown and warrants further evaluation.

The goal of this study is to investigate whether the increased female representation in the POSNA membership roster is reflected at different levels within the organization. The path to leadership positions within POSNA begins with serving as a volunteer member on 1 of the 19 POSNA committees. Therefore, additional analysis was performed to investigate whether there is a gender difference regarding the number of submitted applications among active members to placement to a volunteer committee position. Furthermore, the time to first appointment to the POSNA board of directors (BOD) was analyzed and compared by gender, because this is the next step in the pathway to leadership after committee participation. Lastly, the average time to POSNA presidency from year of membership initiation also was investigated.

METHODS

The membership roster was obtained from POSNA and compared by gender between 2014 and 2018. Leadership and volunteer committee positions were evaluated as published in the annual POSNA committee reference books from 2014 to 2018. Leadership positions were defined as appointment as committee chairs or

council chairs or as election to the BOD or the presidential line (president, president-elect, and vice president).

Members of POSNA are encouraged to apply for open committee positions via the committee appointment program (cap) each year. Applications then are evaluated by the presidential line and respective council chairs and placed into the open positions accordingly after group review. The application process moved from paper to electronic in 2014 and thus subsequent years were evaluated. Applications to the committees available via the CAP system from 2014 to 2018 were compared by gender.

Time to beginning leadership position from the time of membership initiation was analyzed for POSNA presidents and first-time appointment to the BOD for the past 20 years, from 2008 to 2018, and compared by gender.

RESULTS

The membership of POSNA increased from 1199 to 1426 members (24%) from 2014 to 2018. The percentage of women members in POSNA increased from 18% to 22% in the period examined.

Percentage of Women at Each Stage of Pediatric Orthopaedic Society of North America Hierarchy

There was a higher percentage of female CAP applicants (female applicants/total applicants) compared to the percentage of female members in POSNA and the percentage of female volunteers in committees in the years evaluated (Fig. 1). The percentage of female Council and

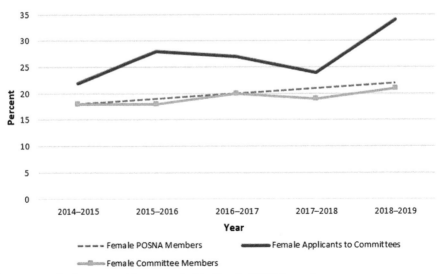

Fig. 1. Percentage of volunteer positions occupied by female POSNA members.

Committee Chairs and the percentage of female members of the BOD in the years evaluated are presented in (Fig. 2). There has been only one woman in the Presidential Line (n = 8) during the period studied (and since the inception of POSNA in 1983).[12]

Proportion of Men and Women in Pediatric Orthopaedic Society of North America Applying to Committees

For every year examined, there was a higher percentage of female POSNA members (number of female CAP applicants/total number of female POSNA members; range 7%–12%) applying for committee positions than male members (5%–9%) (Fig. 3). The average number of applications submitted per female applicant was similar to that of their male counterparts (female: 1.44–2.00 vs male: 1.57–1.86).

Time to Leadership Positions

The time from membership initiation to POSNA presidency was 21 years for the female president. The average number of years from membership initiation to POSNA presidency averaged 19.5 for male presidents (range 14–30 years). The time to first BOD appointment was 8.75 years (SD 4.0) for women and 11.8 years (SD 6.3) for men from the time of initial membership initiation. Total percentage of women on the BOD from 1999 to 2018 was 12.3% (8/65).

DISCUSSION

The percentage of women in POSNA has increased steadily, from 18% in 2014 and to 22% in 2018. There has been a comparable increase in the representation of women volunteering in the committees of POSNA during the same period. The representation of women in the higher levels of the organizational structure of POSNA, however, is lower than the membership percentage. One common rationale for low representation of women in leadership positions is that women are choosing not to participate. Sharkey and colleagues[13] concluded that women in the most active part of their careers participated at significantly lower rates than their male counterparts, as measured by authorship at the annual meetings of POSNA.

To the authors' knowledge, this is the first study to examine female surgeons' national society participation as a benchmark for their overall status and involvement in their field. Specialty society membership often is an important part of a surgeon's career development, and volunteering for society committees is the first step into the leadership ladder of a professional society. The authors' preliminary results show that the women of POSNA are applying for these positions at a higher rate than men. The percentage of women in POSNA applying for volunteer positions is greater than their society membership proportion.

Thus, the shortage of female orthopedic surgeons at the higher levels of POSNA does not correlate, in contrast to the report by Sharkey and colleagues,[13] with decreased involvement at entry-level committee position applications or participation. A possible reason for the decrease in female representation in the BOD and the presidential line may simply be that there is a discernible time lag to advancement to the highest levels of an organization. Analysis of the highest leadership levels of POSNA shows no apparent difference from time of membership initiation to the presidential line or the BOD when compared by gender. Although there are not enough data for statistical calculation, it seems that women ascend the

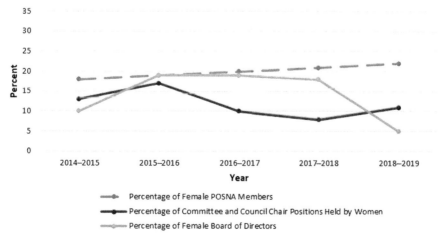

Fig. 2. Percentage of leadership positions occupied by female POSNA members.

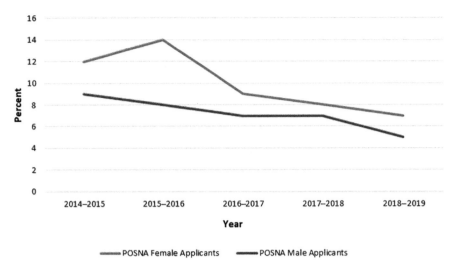

Fig. 3. Percentage of male and female POSNA committee applicants.

leadership ladder at a similar or faster pace than men and, therefore, may indicate that future women leaders are appropriately supported in this organization. Additional research and time are necessary to see whether women will be able to reach equal representation at the highest levels of the organization.

There are several limitations to this study. First, this study is limited to pediatric orthopedic surgeons because the data are from POSNA and may not be generalizable to the rest of orthopedic surgery. In addition, only 5 years of data were available through the POSNA CAP system and the authors' results, therefore, are preliminary. Also, the effect of time lag as related to ascension into a leadership position is unable to be validated in this study but may be able to be reexamined in a future study.

SUMMARY

Female POSNA members apply for committee positions at a greater percentage than do their male counterparts. The authors surmise that the shortage of women in the higher levels of POSNA is not secondary to lack of participation. A likely explanation for the disparity at the highest leadership is because a significant time in the society if required prior to ascending to the BOD or the presidential line. Additional research and time are necessary to see whether the increased volunteerism by women in POSNA will translate into leadership roles in the society.

ACKNOWLEDGMENTS

The authors thank Ms Sharul Saxena, BS, for participating in the technical editing of the article.

REFERENCES

1. Association of American Medical Colleges (AAMC). Active physicians by sex and specialty 2015. Washington, DC. Available at: https://www.aamc.org/data/workforce/reports/458712/1-3-chart.html. Accessed December 3, 2018.
2. Gebhardt MC. Improving diversity in orthopaedic residency programs. J Am Acad Orthop Surg 2007;15(suppl 1):S49–50.
3. Biermann J. Women in orthopaedic surgery residencies in the United States. Acad Med 1998;73: 708–9.
4. Blakemore LC, Hall JM, Biermann JS. Women in surgical residency training programs. J Bone Joint Surg Am 2003;85:2477–80.
5. Association of American Colleges (AAMC). Table B-1: total enrollment by U.S. Medical school and sex, 2014-2015 through 2018-2019. Washington, DC. Available at: https://www.aamc.org/data/facts/enrollmentgraduate/158808/total-enrollment-by-medical-school-by-sex.html. Accessed November 27, 2018.
6. Poon S, Kiridly D, Mutawakkil M, et al. Current trends in sex, race, and ethnic diversity in orthopaedic surgery residency. J Am Acad Orthop Surg 2019. [Epub ahead of print].
7. Okike K, Utuk ME, White AA. Racial and ethnic diversity in orthopaedic surgery residency programs. J Bone Joint Surg Am 2011; 93:e107.
8. Baldwin K, Namdari S, Bowers A, et al. Factors affecting interest in orthopedics among female medical students: prospective analysis. Orthopedics 2011;34:e919–32.
9. Hill JF, Yule A, Zurakowski D, et al. Residents' perceptions of sex diversity in orthopaedic surgery. J Bone Joint Surg Am 2013;95:e1441–6.

10. Poon S, Kiridly D, Brown L, et al. Evaluation of sex, ethnic, and racial diversity across US ACGME-accredited orthopedic subspecialty fellowship programs. Orthopedics 2018;41(5):282–8.

11. Chambers CC, Ihnow SB, Monroe EJ, et al. Women in orthopaedic surgery. J Bone Joint Surg Am 2018; 100(17):e116.

12. Watts HG. A history of the Pediatric Orthopedic Society of North America, 1971 to 1996. 1996. Available at: https://posna.org/POSNA/media/Documents/POSNA_history_book.pdf. Accessed December 18, 2018.

13. Sharkey MS, Feinn RS, Tate VV, et al. Disproportionate participation of males and females in academic pediatric orthopaedics: an analysis of abstract authorship at POSNA 2009-2013. J Pediatr Orthop 2016;36: 433–6.

Racial Diversity in Orthopedic Surgery

Rey N. Ramirez, MD[a],*, Corinna C. Franklin, MD[b]

KEYWORDS

- Diversity • Racial diversity • Ethnic diversity • Representation

KEY POINTS

- African American, Hispanic/Latino, and Native American surgeons are underrepresented in orthopedic surgery.
- Improving diversity would improve patient care through better communication, cultural competency, and improved access.
- Improving diversity would improve the profession by consistently attracting the best medical students and promoting innovation through a diversity of backgrounds and ideas.
- Diversity can be improved through pipeline programs, mentoring, participation in medical schools, and conscious effort.

INTRODUCTION

Most members in the field of orthopedics would agree that there is a lack of diversity. Professional organizations, such as the American Medical Association and the American Academy of Orthopaedic Surgeons (AAOS), have established increased diversity as one of their strategic goals. Examination of the racial and ethnic composition of orthopedic residency programs suggests, however, that this problem is not improving. There are many compelling reasons to believe that better diversity would be beneficial to patients and practices. Based on an analysis of the literature, the authors suggest steps that can be taken to improve diversity in orthopedics.

THE IMPORTANCE OF DIVERSITY

Benefits to Patients

Studies that examine the effect of race consistently demonstrate worse medical outcomes for African Americans and other minorities as compared to white patients. Skinner and colleagues,[1] for example, showed that the number of total knee arthroplasties performed is substantially lower in minority populations. This under-utilization of care persists even after controlling for income. Research persistently shows that ethnic and racial minorities suffer worse outcomes whether in orthopedics[2,3] or other fields. For example, African American patients have significantly worse survival rates for colorectal cancer compared with white patients, regardless of socioeconomic status.[4] Racial minorities also have higher infant mortality rates, have higher total mortality rates, and suffer more serious forms of asthma, diabetes, kidney disease, and heart disease.[5] Although it is likely that multiple variables are involved in this, disparity of care is the 1 variable that can be controlled. Minority physicians currently provide a disproportionate amount of care to medically underserved areas in the United States.[6] Komaromy and colleagues[6] reported that Hispanic/Latino and African American physicians provide care for more uninsured patients and patients with Medicaid insurance than physicians from other groups. The data from their study also demonstrated that despite that patients disproportionately received care from physicians of their own race, only 10% surveyed said that race had been an important factor when choosing their doctor. This suggests that it is not patient

[a] Cooper Medical School of Rowan University, 3 Cooper Plaza, Suite 408, Camden, NJ 08103, USA; [b] Shriners Hospitals for Children, 3551 North Broad Street, Philadelphia, PA 19140, USA
* Corresponding author.
E-mail address: rey.ramirez@gmail.com

Orthop Clin N Am 50 (2019) 337–344
https://doi.org/10.1016/j.ocl.2019.03.010

preference leading to racial matching between physicians and patients.

Minorities also have been shown underrepresented in orthopedic research.[7,8] A systematic review of randomized orthopedic trials showed that randomized trials in orthopedics rarely report data on race or ethnicity and that even when these data are included minority patients are included at numbers substantially lower than expected on the basis of demographics.[7] This study found that only 4.6% of patients were Hispanic/Latino and 6.2% African American.[7] These proportions are 3.5-fold and 2-fold respectively lower than would be expected based on the United States Census.[8] Ethnicity and race must be considered in research while working toward improved treatment and development of implants. For instance, it has been shown that current implants for total knee arthroplasty do not account for the anthropometric features found in some Asian ethnic groups.[9] Increased physician diversity may raise awareness of the differences among various ethnic and racial groups.

Business Will Improve

Improved patient satisfaction is especially important as the era of outcomes-based compensation is entered. Patient-physician communication is an important part of metrics, such as the Consumer Assessment of Healthcare Providers and Systems. Although the authors are not aware of any studies examining the effect of a physician's race directly on these satisfaction measures, there is evidence that diversity improves communication, a key part of these metrics.[10] For example, patients with race-concordant doctors report that they are better able to participate in decision making with their doctor.[11] Minority patients, in general, report worse physician-patient interactions, even after controlling for factors, such as insurance status.[12] A key component of effective communication is cultural competency. This is the ability of providers to deliver health care that recognizes the social, cultural, and linguistic needs of patients. The AAOS has long recognized the need for cultural competency and has attempted to address this need by the creation of a diversity advisory board as well as offering educational resources to educate surgeons on this topic, such as the *Culturally Competent Care Guidebook*, originally published in 2009.[13] There is a positive correlation between cultural competency and patient-perceived quality of patient-physician interactions.[12] Minority physicians are more likely to have cultural competency with minority patients, if for no other reason than that they share similar

life experiences. Because outcomes-based compensation often judges performance of an entire group as well as an individual practitioner, all members in a group will benefit from improved patient satisfaction.

Nonminority physicians also can benefit from the educational value of contact and dialogue among people with different life experiences, outlook, and ideas. For example, surveys of white medical students graduating from medical schools with a more diverse student body show that the students are more prepared to care for patients from minority populations.[14] Furthermore, diversity is attractive in the marketplace. Patients notice the presence of minority providers within a group, and, even if patients of a particular race or ethnicity cannot find a doctor of their own particular heritage, the patients will believe that diversity and cultural competency are generally respected within that group. This feeling of respect attracts new patients, facilitates friendly relations with existing patients, and improves business. Katherine Phillips, of Columbia Business School, summarized it best by stating, "simply interacting with individuals who are different forces group members to prepare better, to anticipate alternative viewpoints, and to expect that reaching consensus will take effort."[15]

These benefits are not theoretic. Numerous studies demonstrate a concrete benefit from increasing diversity. The consulting firm McKinsey published the report "Diversity Matters" in 2015.[16] They showed that "in the United States, there is a linear relationship between racial and ethnic diversity and better financial performance: for every 10% increase in racial and ethnic diversity on the senior-executive team, earnings...rose 0.8%." Companies with high diversity, whether racial, ethnic, or gendered, were more likely to have high financial returns. Conversely, companies with low diversity were more likely to have below-average financial returns. Similar findings were reported by Carter and colleagues,[17] who noted that companies with more diversity (as demonstrated by having women on their board) had improved corporate performance. There also is evidence directly from orthopedics that shows the value of diversity. In the American Society for Surgery of the Hand (ASSH), only 17% of total members belong to underrepresented racial minority groups.[18] They, however, comprise up to 24.8% of attendees and 32.1% of presenters at the annual meeting. This level of engagement shows the value of minority members in the ASSH who are participating at a higher level than their numbers would suggest. Finally, a report by Deloitte showed that employees self-rate their organizations as better able to innovate, more responsive to changing customer needs, and better at team collaboration when the organization is also committed to and supportive of diversity.[19] They further suggest that it is not just diversity but inclusion that matters. To achieve this, orthopedics must begin by changing hiring practices as well as choices for promotion and participation in leadership positions.

Orthopaedic Surgeons Owe It to Ourselves

"Not a good fit"—How often has that critique been heard when evaluating applicants for residency? The Deloitte report highlighted this as a key vulnerable moment that affects the goal of diversity and inclusion.[19] It should be ensured that decisions are made by strict and transparent criteria, wary of unconscious biases. In addition to residency applicants, aspiring medical students will benefit from efforts to improve diversity. A look at the current representation of minorities in orthopedics shows that the participation of most minority groups is far less than demographics suggest.[20] Either minorities are choosing to not go into orthopedics or are not being selected. If the former, then high-quality applicants are being lost to other specialties. Orthopedic surgery is 1 of the most competitive fields, and recruiting the best medical students every year

should be expected; if the best minority candidates are being excluded, that is to the detriment of the specialty. A study by Day and colleagues[21] sheds some light on whether the problem is one of recruitment or exclusion. They compared the racial composition of the applicant pool to that of the orthopedic resident class of 2007 and found no statistically significant variation between the 2 groups. This suggests that minorities are accepted at numbers similar to their application rate. If true, the problem is not attracting minority applicants. The study looked at the results, however, of only 1 year's match. One much older study found that the match rate for underrepresented minorities in 1984 was half of the average.[22] Further research is needed to examine the causes of poor diversity.

THE STATE OF DIVERSITY IN ORTHOPEDICS: WHERE IT IS NOW
Medicine

The United States is an immigrant nation whose population has grown steadily more diverse over time The US Census bureau estimates that in the year 2018 the percentage of the population that is white is 60.7% of the population is white. The Hispanic/Latino share of the population is estimated at 18.1%, whereas African Americans make up 13.4%, Asian Americans 5.8%, and Native Americans 1.3%. Those identifying as mixed race comprise 2.7% of the US

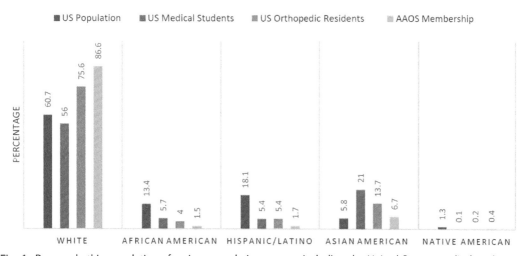

Fig. 1. Race and ethic population of various population groups, including the United States, medical students in the United States, orthopedic residents in the United States, and members of the AAOS. In orthopedic surgery, whites and Asian Americans are overrepresented compared with the general US population, whereas African Americans, Hispanic/Latinos, and Native Americans are under-represented.

population.[8] These numbers continue to change. It is estimated that whites will become a minority by the year 2045.[23]

Although US medical schools' gender composition matches the population fairly closely, their racial diversity does not (Fig. 1). Asian American students are overrepresented in medical school compared with their share of the general US population at 21%. African American students make up only 5.7% of US medical students, and Hispanic/Latino students make up 5.4%. Native Americans are severely underrepresented, even considering their small share of the US population, at 0.1%. White students are slightly underrepresented at 56%.[24] Recent trends show that the diversity in medical schools is not improving. From 2005 to 2014, the total number of medical school graduates increased by 17.4%, whereas the number of African American and Hispanic/Latino graduates decreased by 5.5% and 37.4%, respectively.[25]

Orthopedic Surgery

Orthopedic surgery is even less representative of the racial and ethnic composition of the United States. The most recent AAOS member survey reported that African American surgeons make up just 1.5% of AAOS membership, with Hispanic/Latino members at 1.7% and Asian American members at 6.7%.[26] Orthopedic residency is slightly more diverse. According to the Accreditation Council for Graduate Medical Education (ACGME), in 2016 4% of orthopedic surgery residents were African American, 5.4% were Hispanic/Latino, and 0.2% were Native American. White and Asian American surgeons were overrepresented compared with the general US population at 75.6% and 13.7%, respectively.[27] These numbers show that orthopedic residents are close to being representative of the racial makeup of medical school, if not of US society.

Poon and colleagues[20] recently published a study examining trends in representation in orthopedic residents over the past 10 years. They found that minority representation in orthopedic surgery averaged approximately 25%, lower than any other surgical field. In their study period, representation of Asian American and African American residents remained unchanged, whereas representation of Hispanic/Latino residents increased and that of Native Hawaiian residents decreased.[20] Most concerningly, there was a 32% decrease in minority residents from 2006 to 2015. These trends suggest that, despite efforts, diversity actually may be worsening in orthopedics, although without detailed match numbers, the reasons for this remain unknown.

Subspecialties Within Orthopedics

Unlike the AAOS, the *Pediatric Orthopaedic Society of North America* (POSNA) does not track its members' race or ethnicity. Some guesses may be made based on the ACGME data, because they track participants in ACGME-accredited fellowships. Many pediatric orthopedic fellowships, however, are not ACGME-accredited, so these data can be regarded, at best, as incomplete. Nonetheless, of the 32 pediatric orthopedic fellows listed by the ACGME in 2016, 25 were white (78%), 3 Asian American (9.3%), 2 Hispanic/Latino (6.2%), and 4 unknown (12.5%). None was African American or Native American.[27] Without complete data, it is not possible to determine how the racial percentages of fellows compare to the percentages of applicants of each race.

On the other hand, the ASSH does track the race and ethnicity of its members and those data are available up to 2016. In that year, 83% of United States ASSH members were white, 1.7% African American, 9.8% Asian American, and 4.3% Hispanic/Latino. These numbers represent a shift toward increased racial diversity from 2010, where 92.7% of United States ASSH members were white, 0.9% African American, 4.6% Asian American, and 1.8% Hispanic/Latino.[18]

CURRENT ISSUES RELATED TO DIVERSITY
There Is Much That Is Not Known

There is a lack of data to study diversity in orthopedics. Several organizations do not gather race-related or ethnicity-related data. POSNA, as discussed previously, does not acquire or report data regarding the racial makeup of its membership. The National Resident Matching Program publishes extensive data on match applications and results by location and specialty as well as information on multiple measures as they compare to success in the match (eg, Alpha Omega Alpha membership or US Medical Licensing Examination score). Race or gender, however, is not included in its report. The Association of American Medical Colleges (AAMC) publishes data regarding the race of applicants in orthopedic surgery residencies but does not correlate that with match results.[24] These missing data make it more difficult to assess the full picture of race in orthopedic surgery, particularly as it pertains to success in the match. Given that these numbers can be fairly easily calculated from the results, it is odd that this analysis is omitted.

Worrisome Trends in Diversity in Medical School

A recent article by Abelson and colleagues[25] found that although the total number of graduating medical students increased from 2005 and 2014, the number of African American and Hispanic/Latino students actually decreased. This is despite those groups' overall percentage of the US population increasing during that same interval, meaning that the graduation rate as a percentage of their portion of the population decreased from 59.2% to 46.1% for African American students and from 59.0% to 26.3% for Hispanic/Latino students. Most alarmingly, the number of Hispanic/Latino medical students decreased by 37.4% in that time period. The authors hypothesize that these numbers reflect a decrease in the pipeline of students entering medical school as well as high attrition rates. They also note that some of this discrepancy can be explained by changes in the way the AAMC reports race.

While Orthopedics Stagnate, Other Specialties Improve

Despite these worrisome numbers in medical school, general surgery seems to be making significant gains in diversity. Abelson and colleagues[25] found that despite decreasing representation in medical school, the number of African American and Hispanic/Latino residents in general surgery increased over their study period. African American surgical residents increased 21% in number and 14.8% in percentage and Hispanic/Latino residents increased in number and percentage by 46.7% and 39.1%, respectively. It is not clear why these fields have improved while orthopedics has not.

DIRECTIONS FOR THE FUTURE

What are the barriers to diversity? Broadly speaking, there are several possible causes. One is exclusion, which can be both active and passive. Active discrimination involves direct exclusion of certain groups and passive discrimination involves lack of opportunity for certain groups, such as obtaining a mentor or being chosen to work on a research project. These are key opportunities where great discretion is wielded by existing leaders in orthopedics. These choices influence who does and does not go into orthopedics. A second cause could be that minority medical students find orthopedics less attractive. This seems unlikely given the great interest in obtaining orthopedic residency. In 2018, there were on average 11

applicants for every position.[28] Orthopedic surgeons command among the highest average salary of all medical specialties. Although the lifestyle is demanding, other surgical specialties with similar lifestyles have far greater diversity than orthopedics. It is possible that the current lack of diversity in orthopedics itself is off-putting to minority medical students. Students may not wish to join a field with limited mentors or role models of their own race.

HOW TO INCREASE DIVERSITY

Given the value of diversity, it is desirable to take steps to increase the numbers of orthopedic physicians from minority groups. This view is shared by the AAOS, which has a long-established committee to address diversity. The persistent deficit of minorities of most groups, however, including African American, Hispanic/Latino, and Hawaiian/Pacific Islanders, shows the difficulty of this problem. Again, the percentage of minority residents decreased by more than 30% from 2006 to 2015.[20] Clearly, greater efforts must be made.

Pipeline Programs

Pipeline programs have been shown effective at attracting minorities to orthopedics. A pipeline program works by providing opportunities for exposure, education, and mentoring to potential applicants. It often includes a chance to participate in research. In orthopedics, these programs typically are offered to first-year or second-year medical students and conducted over a summer, although long-term longitudinal programs and short intensive programs also exist. The results from these programs demonstrate their effectiveness.[28,30,32]

One such program is Nth Dimensions.[32] This program is organized into 3 phases. The first consists of Clinical Correlations and Sawbones Bioskills workshops for medical students at historically black colleges and universities. The second involves a summer internship in orthopedics, dermatology, physical therapy, or radiology. The third includes ongoing mentoring and professional development through annual didactics. Over the first 7 years of the program, 118 students participated through phase 2. Minority participants were 15 times more likely (and female participants 50 times more likely) to apply to orthopedic surgery residency than the general medical school population. This program also was effective in helping applicants obtain residency, because 76% of applicants to orthopedics were successful in their match. Another program is the Perry Initiative, which is a pipeline program focused on increasing the number of women in orthopedics. The Perry Initiative conducts single-day outreach programs for female students in both high school and medical school. It recently published reports demonstrating its impact.[30] Three hundred students were involved in the first 3 years of the program, and 30% of participants matched into orthopedics, which is twice the percentage of women in current orthopedic residency classes. Surveys of participants before and after participation showed that the Perry Initiative improved students' perceptions of orthopedics as well as overall interest in the field. Pipeline programs also have proved their effectiveness in other specialties, such as general surgery.[28]

Pipeline programs are supported by volunteers that host students and donors who provide financial support. Information on how to do both is available through the web (www.nthdimensions.org for Nth Dimensions and perryinitiative.org for the Perry Initiative).

Mentoring

These national programs clearly are substantial undertakings and require large investments of time and money. The elements of these programs, however, suggest that smaller measures can be taken by members of the orthopedic community. Mentorship is a key component of these programs. Being a mentor does not require participating in a national program and can be done by minority or nonminority physicians. Mentoring has been shown effective across all fields and encourages students to take the next step in their education.[29] It leads to improved job performance and career advancement.[30] In orthopedics, residents view it as critical to their training.[31] Current orthopedic surgeons can work to provide mentoring to aspiring students. Targeting mentorship to minorities increases the number of applicants to orthopedic residency as well as helps those already in orthopedics rise to leadership positions. These physicians, in turn, will be ideally suited to become mentors to new generations of diverse surgeons. It is incumbent on all interested orthopedic surgeons, however, not just those who belong to minority groups, to provide these mentoring opportunities.

Other Activities to Improve Diversity

Exposure and education also are critical components of pipeline programs. Early exposure to orthopedics in medical school has been shown to increase interest in orthopedics. Although all students are included in orthopedic teaching, underrepresented groups particularly benefit from the exposure.[33,34] Participating in medical school curricula has the added benefit of providing opportunities for students to meet potential mentors. Because the groundwork for application to orthopedic residency must begin early in medical school, it is important that involvement begins in the early years. It is not enough to work with medical students only during their clinical rotations; time must be taken to participate in early coursework, including lectures and small-group teaching.

Program directors are uniquely positioned to affect diversity in their residency programs, beginning with the selection of applicants for interview. At the Johns Hopkins Department of Orthopaedic Surgery, the then-chairman, Dr Richard Stauffer, decided to make the orthopedics program more diverse.[38] This was done without specific policies or quotas. Consideration was given, however, to improving diversity during selection of interviewees. This led to substantial increases in the number of women (from 4% of Hopkins orthopedic residents to 20%) and African Americans (from 0% to 32%). Other organizations have pursued similar strategies, such as the National Football League, whose Rooney Rule policy mandates that teams interview ethnic minority candidates for coaching jobs. Efforts to recruit women and minorities into faculty and leadership positions also can improve diversity. For example, orthopedic programs that have more female faculty members and/or more women in leadership positions are more effective at recruiting female residents.[39] Similar efforts for minority physicians may improve diversity.

Finally, the field of orthopedic surgery must be wary of both active and passive discrimination and make an effort to combat these when encountered. Passive discrimination is more insidious than active discrimination, but this also can be corrected by acknowledging biases and considering whether these biases have an impact on the opportunities given to minorities. Choices are made every day about who gets offered a chance to work on a research project, serve on a committee, or participate in a leadership role. It is important for to consider how these decisions are made.

SUMMARY

There is a clear need for more diversity in orthopedics to improve patient care through better communication, cultural competency, and improved access. It also will improve the profession by consistently attracting the best medical students and promoting innovation through a diversity of backgrounds and ideas. There are many ways to improve diversity, through pipeline programs, mentoring, participation in medical schools, and conscious effort. It is incumbent on all to work to improve representation within orthopedic surgery.

REFERENCES

1. Skinner J, Zhou W, Weinstein J. The influence of income and race on total knee arthroplasty in the United States. J Bone Joint Surg Am 2006;88(10): 2159–66.
2. Cai X, Cram P, Vaughan-Sarrazin M. Are African American patients more likely to receive a total knee arthroplasty in a low-quality hospital? Clin Orthop Relat Res 2012;470(4):1185–93.
3. Ibrahim SA, Stone RA, Han X, et al. Racial/ethnic differences in surgical outcomes in veterans following knee or hip arthroplasty. Arthritis Rheum 2005;52(10):3143–51.
4. Wudel LJ, Chapman WC, Shyr Y, et al. Disparate outcomes in patients with colorectal cancer: effect of race on long-term survival. Arch Surg 2002; 137(5):550–6. Available at: http://www.ncbi.nlm. nih.gov/pubmed/11982467.
5. Lancet T. Ending racial and ethnic health disparities in the USA. Lancet 2011;377(9775):1379.
6. Komaromy M, Grumbach K, Drake M, et al. The role of black and hispanic physicians in providing health care for underserved populations. N Engl J Med 1996;334(20):1305–10.
7. Somerson JS, Bhandari M, Vaughan CT, et al. Lack of diversity in orthopaedic trials conducted in the United States. J Bone Joint Surg Am 2014; 96(e56):1–6.
8. United States Census Bureau. United States census quick facts. 2010. Available at: https://www.census. gov/quickfacts/fact/table/US/PST045217. Accessed August 2, 2019.
9. Chung BJ, Kang JY, Kang YG, et al. Clinical implications of femoral anthropometrical features for total knee arthroplasty in Koreans. J Arthroplasty 2015; 30(7):1220–7.
10. Reede JY. A recurring theme: the need for minority physicians. Health Aff 2003;22(4):91–3.
11. Cooper-Patrick L, Gallo JJ, Gonzales JJ, et al. Race, gender, and partnership in the patient-physician relationship. JAMA 1999;282(6):583–9.
12. Arbelaez JJ, Cooper LA, Saha S. Patient-physician relationships and racial disparities in the quality of health care. Am J Public Health 2003;93(10): 1713–9.
13. Jimenez RL, Lewis VO. Culturally Competent Care Guidebook. AAOS; 2009.
14. Saha S, Guiton G, Wimmers PF, et al. Student body racial and ethnic composition and diversity-related outcomes in US medical schools. JAMA 2008; 300(10):1135–45.
15. Phillips, Katherine W. How diversity makes us smarter. Scientific American 2014;311(4):43–7.
16. Hunt V, Layton D, Prince S. McKinsey & Company: Diversity matters 2015;15–29.
17. Carter NM, Joy L, Wagner HM, et al. The bottom line: corporate performance and women's representation on boards. Catalyst 2004. https://doi. org/10.1037/e514402010-001.
18. Earp BE, Mora AN, Rozental TD. Extending a hand: increasing diversity at the American society for surgery of the hand. J Hand Surg Am 2018;43(7): 649–56.
19. Bourke J, Dillon B. Waiter, is that inclusion in my soup? A new recipe to improve business performance. Deloitte 2013.
20. Poon S, Kiridly D, Mutawakkil M, et al. Current trends in sex, race, and ethnic diversity in orthopaedic surgery residency. J Am Acad Orthop Surg 2019;1–9. https://doi.org/10.5435/JAAOS-D-18-00131.
21. Day CS, Lage DE, Ahn CS. Diversity based on race, ethnicity, and sex between academic orthopaedic surgery and other specialties: a comparative study. J Bone Joint Surg Am 2010;92(13): 2328–35.
22. Jordan WC. Success of minority applicants in the National Residency Matching Program. J Natl Med Assoc 1986;78(8):737–9.
23. National population projections tables. United States Census Bureau 2017. Available at: www. census.gov. Accessed February 9, 2019.
24. Table A-9: matriculants to U.S. medical schools by race, selected combinations of race/ethnicity and sex, 2015-2016 through 2018-2019. Assoc Am Med Coll. 2018. Available at: https://www.aamc.org/ download/321474/data/factstablea9.pdf. Accessed November 9, 2018.
25. Abelson JS, Symer MM, Yeo HL, et al. Surgical time out: our counts are still short on racial diversity in academic surgery. Am J Surg 2018; 215(4):542–8.
26. AAOS Department of Research Quality and Scientific Affairs. Orthopaedic practice in the US 2016 2011. Rosemont (IL): American Academy of Orthopaedic Surgeons; 2011.
27. Brotherton SE, Etzel SI. Graduate medical education, 2016-2017. JAMA 2012;318(23):2368–87.
28. Butler PD, Britt LD, Richard CE, et al. The diverse surgeons' initiative: longitudinal assessment of a successful national program. J Am Coll Surg 2015; 220(3):362–9.

29. Dubois DL, Holloway BE, Valentine JC, et al. Effectiveness of mentoring programs for youth : a meta-analytic review. Am J Community Psychol 2002; 30(2):157–97.

30. Lattanza LL, Meszaros-Dearolf L, O'Connor MI, et al. The Perry Initiative's Medical Student Outreach Program Recruits Women Into Orthopaedic Residency. Clin Orthop Relat Res 2016;474(9):1962–6.

31. Flint JH, Jahangir AA, Browner BD, et al. The value of mentorship in orthopaedic surgery resident education: the residents' perspective. J Bone Joint Surg Am 2009;91:1017–22.

32. Mason BS, Ross W, Ortega G, et al. Can a strategic pipeline initiative increase the number of women and underrepresented minorities in orthopaedic surgery? Clin Orthop Relat Res 2016;474(9): 1979–85.

33. Baldwin KD, Namdari S, Keenan MA, et al. Factors affecting interest in orthopedics among female medical students: a prospective analysis. Orthopedics 2011. https://doi.org/10.3928/01477447-20111021-17.

34. Bernstein J, Dicaprio MR, Mehta S. The relationship between required medical school instruction in musculoskeletal medicine and application rates to orthopaedic surgery residency programs. J Bone Joint Surg Am 2004; 86(10):2335–8.

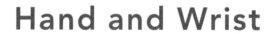

Hand and Wrist

Wrist Denervation
Techniques and Outcomes

Chia H. Wu, MD, MBA, Robert J. Strauch, MD*

KEYWORDS

- Wrist denervation • Denervation • Wrist pain • Wrist arthritis • Radiocarpal arthritis

KEY POINTS

- Wrist denervation is a safe and effective procedure that can ameliorate wrist pain secondary to a variety of pathologic conditions, including degenerative and posttraumatic causes.
- Wrist denervation does not preclude traditional salvage procedures, such as partial or complete wrist fusions or proximal row carpectomy.
- Although theoretically possible, sequelae such as Charcot joints have neither been reported nor have been observed after wrist denervation.

INTRODUCTION

Chronic pain of the wrist can be attributed to multiple causes, including posttraumatic and degenerative causes. Over time, it can become debilitating and cause dysfunction for patients. Ideally, orthopedic procedures are designed to correct or restore anatomy in order to achieve pain relief. As a last resort, salvage procedures, such as arthrodesis or resection, may be required.

An alternative to wrist salvage procedures is wrist denervation. Because pain is transmitted by nerves that innervate the wrist joint, transecting these articular nerve branches reduces pain without causing motor or sensory deficits. To the authors' knowledge, Charcot joints have never been reported following wrist denervation, as complete wrist denervation is not possible with existing procedures.

Hilton's law, described by Dr John Hilton, a British anatomist and surgeon, states that nerves crossing a joint give off branches to innervate that joint. As such, it logically follows that cutting these articular branches can reduce pain, as proposed by Dr Camitz in 1933, initially for treatment of osteoarthritis of the hip. Since then, Tavernier reported excellent results in 75% of patients

undergoing hip joint denervation in 1949. In 1954, Marcacci proposed denervating knee joints, while Nyakas and Kiss expanded the indications to the ankle, tarsal joints, and shoulder.[1]

However, it was not until 1959 that Dr Albrecht Wilhelm[1-3] first described and performed wrist joint denervation for arthritis in a patient with a scaphoid nonunion. Subsequently, this technique has been replicated and modified by many surgeons with good outcomes.[4-19] Dr Wilhelm and several other investigators intended the procedure to be "complete," or "total," denervation, by transecting all of the known articular branches. In 2002, Weinstein and Berger[15] reported good results with transection of solely the posterior and anterior interosseous articular nerve branches. Dellon and colleagues,[8] on the other hand, reported good results with transecting only the anterior interosseous nerve (AIN).

Classic descriptions of wrist denervation involve multiple small incisions. The AIN is located on the distal aspect of pronator quadratus and is transected via cauterization. Weinstein and Berger[15] first described transecting just the posterior interosseous nerve (PIN) and AIN through a longitudinal dorsal incision as a "partial" wrist denervation.

Disclosure Statement: The authors do not have any commercial or financial conflict of interest.

New York Presbyterian–Columbia University Medical Center, 622 West, 168th Street PH 11-1119, New York City, NY 10032, USA

* Corresponding author.

E-mail address: rjs8@cumc.columbia.edu

Orthop Clin N Am 50 (2019) 345–356

https://doi.org/10.1016/j.ocl.2019.03.002

The authors' current preference for wrist denervation typically performed for dorsal and radial wrist pain uses a modification of Berger's approach to transect the PIN and AIN. Through the same dorsal incision, branches of the superficial radial and ulnar nerves may also be removed. If the patient complains of significant pain on the radial side of the wrist joint (eg, scapholunate advanced collapse [SLAC] wrist), a volar longitudinal incision can be used to transect branches of the lateral antebrachial cutaneous nerve (LABCN) running longitudinally from the radial vascular bundle to the joint, in addition to allowing easier access to the more volar branches of the superficial branch of radial nerve (SBRN), sending articular twigs down to the joint. This technique ensures that the radial side of the wrist is free of any articular branches from the superficial radial and LABCNs. If the patient also has ulnar-sided wrist pain, a constant articular branch leading to the triangular fibrocartilage complex (TFCC) area from the dorsal sensory branch of the ulnar nerve may also be included in the denervation procedure.

NEUROANATOMY

Although many nerve branches have been described as innervating the wrist joint, there are 3 of particular relevance to this procedure:

1. The median nerve does not provide any known articular branches directly as it travels across the wrist into the carpal tunnel. It innervates the joint via its AIN and palmar cutaneous nerve branches.
2. The ulnar nerve innervates the ulnar wrist via a branch from the dorsal sensory ulnar nerve as well as branches from the deep motor branch of the ulnar nerve, which is located in the region of the hook of hamate. Other smaller articular branches pass through the intermetacarpal spaces and emerge dorsally to innervate the carpometacarpal joints of the index to small fingers.
3. The radial nerve innervates the wrist joint through the PIN and small branches arising from the radial sensory nerve. Other relevant nerves in this location include the LABCN, which can be found running longitudinally, accompanying the radial artery and venae comitantes. In addition, small branches from the posterior and medial antebrachial cutaneous nerves may provide articular innervation, but these are not typically included in the denervations the authors perform.

PREOPERATIVE DIAGNOSTIC INJECTIONS

Although Weinstein and Berger[15] did not find a correlation between the results of preoperative diagnostic PIN/AIN nerve blocks and ultimate postoperative pain relief or disabilities of the arm, shoulder, and hand (DASH) scores, some investigators advocate its use.[4–6] In the authors' experience, they have not found preoperative anesthetic injections helpful in predicting postoperative pain relief.

INDICATIONS

The ideal candidate is a skeletally mature patient with a chronic, painful radiocarpal or ulnocarpal wrist condition, causing sufficient wrist pain to warrant a surgical procedure after exhausting nonoperative treatment.

The senior author will frequently perform denervation as a stand-alone procedure; however, resection of the PIN has occasionally been performed in adolescents when undergoing concomitant excision of a dorsal ganglion cyst with good response. In addition, adolescents requiring surgery for Kienbock disease may also benefit from concomitant denervation in the authors' experience. There is no upper age limit for this procedure.

Wrist denervation can be used as an adjunct procedure or as a stand-alone procedure. Indications typically include arthritis due to previous trauma, SLAC, or SNAC (scaphoid nonunion advanced collapse) wrist, and Kienbock disease among other wrist disorders.

Theoretically, denervation can be undertaken for any painful wrist condition before embarking on salvage procedures. Isolated causes of ulnar-sided wrist pain (eg, triangular fibrocartilage tears) have not been treated with a stand-alone wrist denervation, but denervation may serve as an adjunct procedure. In this way, wrist denervation can be an alternative to salvage procedures, such as partial or complete wrist fusions, proximal row carpectomy, and total wrist arthroplasty.

Because wrist denervation as a primary procedure is performed for chronic wrist pain, the painful condition typically needs to be present for at least 6 months to a year and having failed nonoperative treatment before consideration of surgery. Denervation is frequently combined with other procedures as a method of treating current pain or alleviating future wrist pain (eg, ganglion excisions, wrist fractures). The denervation procedure does not "burn any bridges." It is also recommended that the surgeon discuss salvage procedures with the patient pre-operatively in case that wrist denervation does not provide sufficient pain relief.

CONTRAINDICATIONS

Absolute contraindications to denervation are active infection, cognitive impairment, or poor compliance. Correctable wrist conditions, such as scaphoid nonunion without significant arthritis, should be treated by addressing the underlying problem. Relative contraindications to wrist denervation include diffuse arthritis, such as those seen secondary to severe rheumatoid arthritis, or pain that is nonanatomic, such as diffuse distal forearm pain (denervation can only alleviate pain downstream from the site of nerve transection). Preoperative counseling is especially important because patients desiring a definitive operation (eg, arthrodesis) with a minimal chance of revision may prefer complete wrist arthrodesis, particularly if there is limited preoperative wrist motion.

SURGICAL TECHNIQUE

Classically, Dr Wilhelm's original technique[1] included transecting up to 10 articular nerve branches for a successful wrist denervation, which called for the use of 5 small incisions, including cauterization of PIN through a transverse dorsal incision. He preferred a curvilinear incision extending from the trapezium to the flexor surface of the distal radius in order to remove articular fibers from the LABCN, superficial radial nerve, palmar cutaneous branch of the median nerve, and AIN. A separate curved incision about the ulnar head is made to denervate articular fibers of the dorsal sensory branch of the ulnar nerve.

This procedure can be performed with standard hand surgery instrumentation, loupe magnification, and a bipolar cautery in a supine position on a hand table. Isolated PIN and AIN denervation via a single dorsal longitudinal incision can usually be done with local anesthesia and sedation. If an additional longitudinal volar incision is required, then regional or general anesthesia may be preferred.

AUTHORS' PREFERRED TECHNIQUE
Dorsal Incision and Dissection

If the procedure is performed as a primary procedure, both dorsal and volar longitudinal incisions are recommended to ensure pain relief (**Fig. 1**). When performed in conjunction with other dorsal wrist procedures, such as dorsal

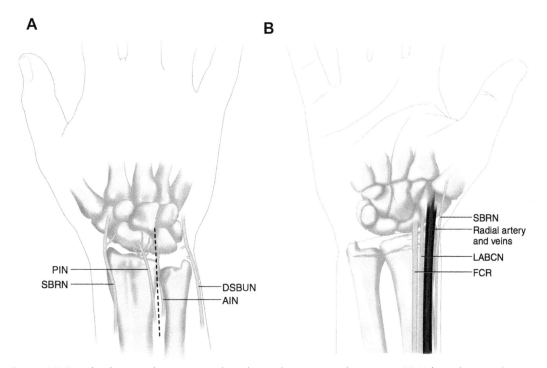

Fig. 1. (*A*) Dorsal right wrist showing nerve branches with respect to the incision. (*B*) Volar right wrist showing flexor carpi radialis (FCR), radial artery, and nerve branches involved. (*Adapted from* Strauch RJ. Denervation of the wrist joint for chronic pain. In: Slutsky DJ, editor. Principles and practice of wrist surgery, 1st edition. Philadelphia: Saunders; 2010; with permission.)

ganglion excision, or with salvage wrist operations, a more limited denervation is usually sufficient. It is the authors' preference to not routinely transect the ulnar-sided nerve branches from the dorsal sensory branch of ulnar nerve (DSBUN) unless significant preoperative ulnar wrist pain is present.

The longitudinal dorsal incision is centered above the distal radioulnar joint, extending approximately 3 to 5 cm proximally. The interval between the extensor digitorum communis (EDC) and the extensor digiti minimi (EDM) is used (**Figs. 2** and **3**). The extensor tendons should be carefully protected with retractors.

1. PIN localization: The EDC is retracted radially, and the PIN is identified on the floor of the fourth dorsal compartment (**Fig. 4**). The PIN is found to be on average 0.87 mm in diameter and is equally likely to be radial or ulnar to the posterior interosseous artery.[20] One to 2 cm of the PIN is resected carefully using bipolar cautery to minimize neuroma formation postoperatively (**Figs. 5** and **6**). It should be noted that the posterior interosseous artery

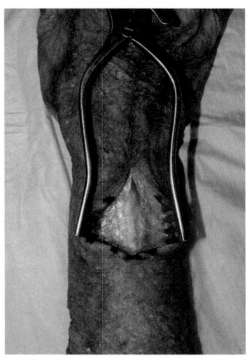

Fig. 3. Interval between the EDC and the EDM retracted out of the way on either side of the incision. (*From* Strauch RJ. Denervation of the wrist joint for chronic pain. In: Slutsky DJ, editor. Principles and practice of wrist surgery, 1st edition. Philadelphia: Saunders; 2010; with permission.)

will be found running alongside PIN and should be preserved.

2. AIN localization: This nerve is found volar to the interosseous membrane. The membrane is incised, exposing the dorsal surface of the pronator quadratus muscle (**Fig. 7**). The AIN is usually located ulnar to the PIN and is radial to the anterior interosseous artery 80% of the time. The average AIN diameter is 1.5 mm at the proximal end of the incision. It gives off about 4 motor branches, with the largest one being the most proximal branch. The first branch is found at about 4 cm proximal to the ulnar head. The distal sensory branch, which is the branch that is transected, is typically about 0.6 mm in diameter. In 40% of cases, there is a 0.4-mm branch to the distal radioulnar joint as well. Therefore, a 1-cm resection of the AIN at a level no further than 2 cm proximal to the ulnar head should denervate sensory branches without denervating the pronator quadratus muscle.[20–22] Occasionally, the AIN can prove elusive, but careful spreading dissection through the pronator quadratus will reveal its position (**Fig. 8**).

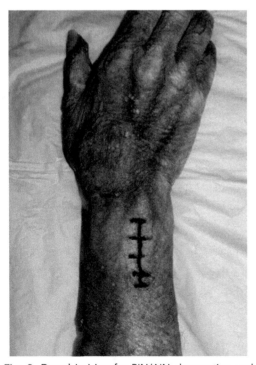

Fig. 2. Dorsal incision for PIN/AIN denervation and DSBUN denervation. (*From* Strauch RJ. Denervation of the wrist joint for chronic pain. In: Slutsky DJ, editor. Principles and practice of wrist surgery, 1st edition. Philadelphia: Saunders; 2010; with permission.)

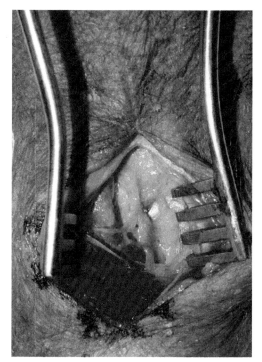

Fig. 4. The EDC is retracted radially, revealing the PIN. (*From* Strauch RJ. Denervation of the wrist joint for chronic pain. In: Slutsky DJ, editor. Principles and practice of wrist surgery, 1st edition. Philadelphia: Saunders; 2010; with permission.)

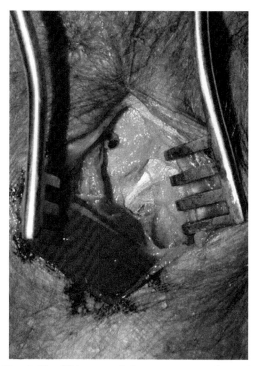

Fig. 6. The PIN resected. Interosseous membrane is visible. (*From* Strauch RJ. Denervation of the wrist joint for chronic pain. In: Slutsky DJ, editor. Principles and practice of wrist surgery, 1st edition. Philadelphia: Saunders; 2010; with permission.)

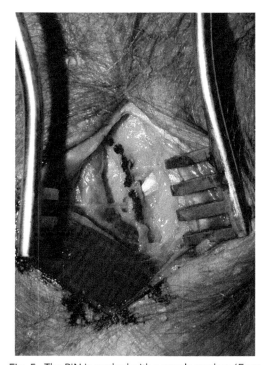

Fig. 5. The PIN is marked with a purple marker. (*From* Strauch RJ. Denervation of the wrist joint for chronic pain. In: Slutsky DJ, editor. Principles and practice of wrist surgery, 1st edition. Philadelphia: Saunders; 2010; with permission.)

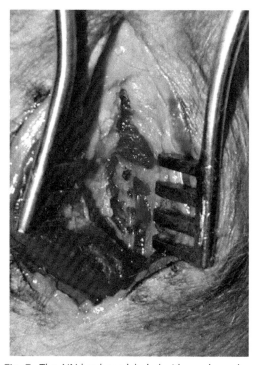

Fig. 7. The AIN has been labeled with purple marker. (*From* Strauch RJ. Denervation of the wrist joint for chronic pain. In: Slutsky DJ, editor. Principles and practice of wrist surgery, 1st edition. Philadelphia: Saunders; 2010; with permission.)

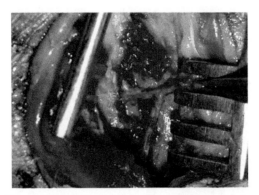

Fig. 8. The AIN branches to the pronator quadratus are preserved, and distal resection of the nerve is performed. (*From* Strauch RJ. Denervation of the wrist joint for chronic pain. In: Slutsky DJ, editor. Principles and practice of wrist surgery, 1st edition. Philadelphia: Saunders; 2010; with permission.)

3. Superficial radial nerve: Articular branches from the SBRN can be found leading down to the wrist joint in the plane between the fascia and the skin. From the dorsal incision, the authors recommend carefully sweeping radially and bluntly in this plane to locate small sensory branches that can run with small vessels and appear vascular. These are coagulated with the bipolar cautery, taking care to stay well away from the proper SBRN branches.

4. DSBUN: From the same dorsal incision, dissection is carried bluntly and ulnarly at a level between the skin and the fascia. At the volar aspect of the ulna, a branch from the DSBUN is found heading toward the region of the TFCC, which may be coagulated with the bipolar if desired (**Figs. 9** and **10**). Alternatively, an additional incision can be made superficial to the sixth compartment to dissect out the DSBUN if adequate visualization cannot be achieved from the dorsal incision, but this is usually not necessary.

Volar Incision and Dissection

If desired, a longitudinal volar incision about 2.5 cm in length is made overlying the radial artery (**Fig. 11**). From this incision, the following nerves can be accessed:

1. Superficial radial nerve: Dissection proceeds at the level between skin and fascia to allow for cauterization of remaining superficial nerves. Additional small vascular-looking branches from the superficial radial nerve may be identified and coagulated (**Fig. 12**). The skin flap connecting the dorsal and

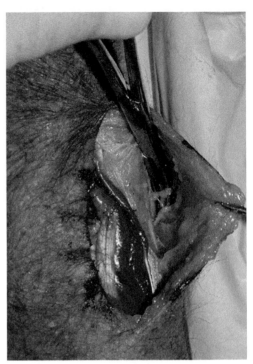

Fig. 9. Ulnar dissection identifies the branch to the TFCC area from the dorsal sensory branch of the ulnar nerve. (*From* Strauch RJ. Denervation of the wrist joint for chronic pain. In: Slutsky DJ, editor. Principles and practice of wrist surgery, 1st edition. Philadelphia: Saunders; 2010; with permission.)

volar incisions can be completely elevated in this manner, and all small nerve branches running down to the joint from the SBRN can be eliminated.

2. LABCN: These 2 tiny nerve branches can be found running with the radial artery and veins and transected as described by Wilhelm.[1–3] These branches can frequently be mistaken for venae comitantes accompanying the radial artery, but are clearly distinct when meticulous dissection has been carried out (**Fig. 13**). In practice, this technique has occasionally caused a painful Tinel sign over that area postoperatively, and as such, the authors now recommend isolating the radial artery and venae comitantes as they course across the wrist joint with a vessiloop and transecting the small articular nerve branches from the LABCN leading down into the joint with bipolar cautery instead of transecting the longitudinally running LABCN branches alongside the vessels.

3. Palmar cutaneous branch of the median nerve: The palmar cutaneous nerve is usually not dissected out separately out of concern for neuroma formation (**Fig. 14**).

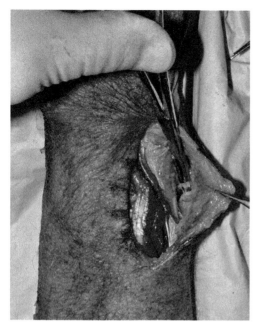

Fig. 10. Clamp showing the articular branches of the dorsal sensory branch of the ulnar nerve. (*From* Strauch RJ. Denervation of the wrist joint for chronic pain. In: Slutsky DJ, editor. Principles and practice of wrist surgery, 1st edition. Philadelphia: Saunders; 2010; with permission.)

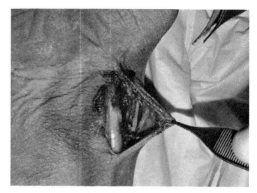

Fig. 12. Sensory branch of the radial nerve branches to the joint seen via volar incision. (*From* Strauch RJ. Denervation of the wrist joint for chronic pain. In: Slutsky DJ, editor. Principles and practice of wrist surgery, 1st edition. Philadelphia: Saunders; 2010; with permission.)

In the authors' experience, the AIN and PIN are distinct nerves that are readily identifiable. They should be positively identified every time. The other nerve branches are tiny and may appear as small vessels. A headlight is quite helpful to look under the skin flap connecting the 2 incisions. The authors recommend interrupted simple 5-0 nylon sutures for closure. Subcutaneous or subdermal sutures are not necessary.

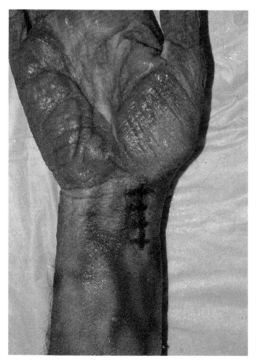

Fig. 11. Volar incision marked on the skin. (*From* Strauch RJ. Denervation of the wrist joint for chronic pain. In: Slutsky DJ, editor. Principles and practice of wrist surgery, 1st edition. Philadelphia: Saunders; 2010; with permission.)

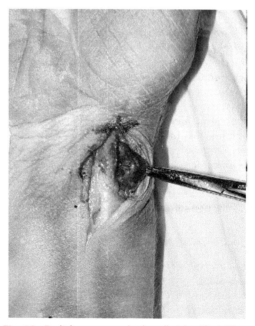

Fig. 13. Radial neurovascular bundle identified. (*From* Strauch RJ. Denervation of the wrist joint for chronic pain. In: Slutsky DJ, editor. Principles and practice of wrist surgery, 1st edition. Philadelphia: Saunders; 2010; with permission.)

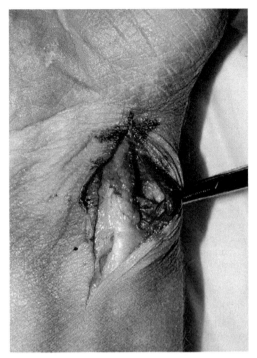

Fig. 14. Radial neurovascular bundle isolated and articular nerve branches from LABCN transected. (*From* Strauch RJ. Denervation of the wrist joint for chronic pain. In: Slutsky DJ, editor. Principles and practice of wrist surgery, 1st edition. Philadelphia: Saunders; 2010; with permission.)

POSTOPERATIVE CARE

A fiberglass volar wrist splint is applied in the operating room. Finger motion is encouraged immediately. Sutures are removed at the first postoperative visit, typically 10 to 14 days after surgery. A new wrist splint is placed for an additional 2 weeks to be worn full time except when showering. Immobilization of the wrist for 1 month postoperatively is helpful. Thereafter, wrist range of motion and return to activities are unrestricted. Patients should be counseled that the volar incision can be tender for several months, and that the full benefit of the surgery may not be realized for up to 6 months.

COMPLICATION AND CONTROVERSIES

Many investigators transect the AIN and PIN as a stand-alone procedure, without performing a more extensive denervation. It is not possible to completely denervate the wrist because there are many tiny unnamed nerve branches. The authors recommend the previously described technique after trying multiple variations of the surgical techniques. The only branches that are missed by this technique are the dorsal sensory branch of the ulnar nerve that perforates the intermetacarpal spaces, and some articular branches of the palmar cutaneous branch of the median nerve as well as twigs from the motor branch of the ulnar nerve. In the case of insufficient pain relief postoperatively after 8 to 12 months, salvage operations may be performed. Salvage procedures should not be considered a complication but rather part of the informed risk-benefit tradeoff when the patient agreed to the procedure. Transient paresthesias from retraction have been observed as well as some neuritic symptoms (focal Tinel) for up to 6 months after resecting the lateral antebrachial nerve branches. As such, the authors no longer recommend resecting these branches, as noted above.

RESULTS

It is the authors' experience that limited denervation of AIN and PIN in addition to the branches of the LABCN and SBRN will be satisfactory in most patients, as advocated and corroborated by other investigators.[23,24] It is important to note, however, that variations in technique do exist. Limited denervation involving the AIN only has been described.[8] Ferreres and colleagues[12] demonstrated that pain relief of a stand-alone PIN neurectomy tended to deteriorate over time when compared with a classic Wilhelm denervation. The literature also lacks consensus on whether preoperative injections reliably predict postoperative pain relief,[4–6,15] and the authors do not perform them preoperatively.

Buck-Gramcko[5] was the first to report pain relief in two-thirds of the patients who underwent the procedure in 1977. In 1984, Dellon and colleagues[8] reported good results with just transection of the AIN. More recently, multiple retrospective studies with up to 12-year follow-up have replicated good clinical results with wrist denervation in the young military and middle-aged civilian population.[25] In fact, 1 systematic review found that even isolated PIN transection can be effective in dorsal wrist pain relief.[26] It should be noted that there are no published prospective studies or randomized controlled trials published on this topic to the authors' knowledge.

As seen in **Table 1**, multiple studies, starting with the study by Dr Wilhelm in the 1960s, have reported good to excellent pain relief in 60% to 90% of the patients. More recently, Braga-Silva and colleagues[19] reported maintenance of 80% pain relief at 6-year follow-up, in

Table 1
Results from selected published studies

Author, y (Country)	Technique	No. of Patients	Average Follow-Up (y)	Results
Wilhelm,[3] 1966 (Germany)	Wilhelm	21	1.5	80% good or excellent
Geldmacher et al,[4] 1972 (Germany)	Wilhelm	35	Not given	72% good or excellent
Buck-Gramcko,[5] 1977 (Germany)	Wilhelm	102 (own cases)	3	66% good and satisfactory
Buck-Gramcko,[5] 1977 (Germany) reported at German Hand Society	Wilhelm	195	3	66% good and satisfactory
Rostlund et al,[7] 1980 (Sweden)	Modified Wilhelm	9	1.8	90% "improved considerably"
Dellon et al,[8] 1984 (US)	AIN only	12	1	92% good to excellent
Ishida et al,[10] 1993 (Japan)	Wilhelm (with preoperative nerve blocks)	29	4.3	24% satisfied; Total denervation better results than partial
Ferreres et al,[12] 1995 (France and Spain)	Wilhelm vs PIN alone	22 total vs 30 PIN alone	Total: 5.4, Partial: 4.7	Total denervation: 86% good to excellent; PIN only: results worsened by 1 y
Grechenig et al,[13] 1998 (Austria)	Wilhelm	22	4.2	77% good to excellent
Wilhelm,[1] 2001 (Germany)	Wilhelm	374	Variable	At 1.2 y: 81% good to excellent; at 2.2 y: 77.8% good to excellent; at 10.5 y: 62.5% good to excellent
Weinstein & Berger,[15] 2002 (US)	AIN and PIN only	19	2.5	85% reported satisfied
Rothe et al,[16] 2006 (Germany)	Wilhelm	46	6.2	62.5 good to very good
Schweizer et al,[17] 2006 (Switzerland)	Wilhelm	70	9.6	66% report long-term improvement; 50% complete or substantial pain relief
Van de Pol et al,[18] 2006 (Netherlands)	Modified Wilhelm: 1 dorsal and volar longitudinal incision	Technique only		
Hofmeister et al,[23] 2006 (US)	AIN and PIN only (Berger technique)	48 (50 wrists)	2.3	Statistically significant improvement in grip strength; statistically sign; improvement in pain relief (0–100 scale) & DASH

(continued on next page)

Author, y (Country)	Technique	No. of Patients	Average Follow-Up (y)	Results
Strauch,[27] 2010 (US)	Modified Berger	8	1.5	75% reported excellent results; 1 patient was later diagnosed with rheumatoid arthritis; 1 patient had severe SLAC wrist
Braga-Silva et al,[19] 2011 (Brazil)	Wilhelm	49	Minimum of 6 y	80% reported improvement in pain at 1 y; improvement in grip strength maintained at 6 y; improvement in range of motion in all 3 axes
Delclaux et al,[25] 2017 (France)	Modified Wilhelm	33	8	75% reduction in pain on VAS; no change in wrist motion or strength; osteoarthritis progression in 6 patients
Vanden Berge et al,[26] 2017 (US)	PIN only	136	4.3	Systematic review; 89% able to return to work; 26% had recurrence of pain at 12.3 mo postoperatively
Fuchsberger et al,[28] 2018 (Germany)	Wilhelm	375	12.2	Pain reduction of 52%; 68% of patients experience pain relief; 44% experience complete relief at last follow-up
O'Shaughnessy et al,[29] 2018 (US)	Berger	89	6.8	69% did not undergo additional procedure during study period; average Mayo wrist score improved from 48 to 77
Sgromolo et al,[30] 2018 (US)	Berger	13	1	In active military population; improved pain score from 4 to 2.2; range of motion unchanged

Adapted from Strauch RJ. Denervation of the wrist joint for chronic pain. In: Slutsky DJ, editor. Principles and practice of wrist surgery, 1st edition. Philadelphia: Saunders; 2010; with permission.

accordance with the results the authors published in 2010.[27] The authors now counsel patients that they can expect a maximum of approximately 80% pain relief, and that although the pain will not be completely gone, this procedure is motion preserving and does not preclude later definitive salvage procedures if needed. The possibility of a Charcot wrist is merely theoretical and has not been reported since the procedure's initial description by Wilhelm in 1966. In fact, new biomechanical evidence suggests that there is no change in proprioception after partial wrist denervation.[31]

Postoperatively, the authors typically recommend immobilization in a splint for 1 month before beginning range of motion. Patient may not experience maximum pain relief from the procedure until 6 months after surgery.[27]

SUMMARY

Wrist denervation is an effective procedure that treats the symptoms of pain without altering the underlying bony anatomy or reducing motion. Theoretically, severing C fibers to remove the pain sensation can cause a Charcot joint, but this has never been reported or observed in the literature or in the authors' experience.[1] As this procedure gains more traction, it is possible that the use of denervation as a treatment concept may be expanded to other areas of hand surgery in the near future, as exemplified in its use in the case thumb carpometacarpal joint arthritis.[32]

Overall, the authors believe this is an effective, safe, and biologically friendly procedure that has minimum downside that should be considered whenever appropriate for management of chronic wrist pain.

REFERENCES

1. Wilhelm A. Denervation of the wrist. Tech Hand Up Extrem Surg 2001;5(1):14–30.
2. Wilhelm A. Denervation of the wrist. Hefte Unfallheilkd 1965;81:109–14.
3. Wilhelm A. Articular denervation and its anatomical foundation. A new therapeutic principle in hand surgery. On the treatment of the later stages of lunatomalacia and navicular pseudoarthrosis. Hefte Unfallheilkd 1966;86:1–109 [in German].
4. Geldmacher J, Legal HR, Brug E. Results of denervation of the wrist and wrist joint by Wilhelm's method. Hand 1972;4:57–9.
5. Buck-Gramcko D. Denervation of the wrist joint. J Hand Surg Am 1977;2:54–61.
6. Dellon AL, Seif SS. Anatomic dissections relating the posterior interosseous nerve to the carpus and the etiology of dorsal wrist ganglion pain. J Hand Surg Am 1978;3:326–32.
7. Rostlund T, Somnier F, Axelsson R. Denervation of the wrist: an alternative in conditions of chronic pain. Acta Orthop Scand 1980;51:609–16.
8. Dellon AL, Mackinnon SE, Daneshvar A. Terminal branch of anterior interosseous nerve as source of wrist pain. J Hand Surg Br 1984;9:316–22.
9. Fukumoto K, Kojima T, Kinoshita Y, et al. An anatomic study of the innervation of the wrist joint and Wilhelm's technique for denervation. J Hand Surg Am 1993;18:484–9.
10. Ishida O, Tsai TM, Atasoy E. Long-term results of denervation of the wrist joint for chronic wrist pain. J Hand Surg Br 1993;18:76–80.
11. Ferreres A, Suso S, Ordi J, et al. Wrist denervation: anatomical considerations. J Hand Surg Br 1995;20:761–8.
12. Ferreres A, Suso S, Foucher G, et al. Wrist denervation: surgical considerations. J Hand Surg Br 1995;20:769–72.
13. Grechenig W, Mahring M, Clement HG. Denervation of the radiocarpal joint. J Bone Joint Surg Br 1998;80:504–7.
14. Ferreres A, Foucher G, Suso S. Extensive denervation of the wrist. Tech Hand Up Extrem Surg 2002;6(1):36–41.
15. Weinstein LP, Berger RA. Analgesic benefit, functional outcome and patient satisfaction after partial wrist denervation. J Hand Surg Am 2002;27:833–9.
16. Rothe M, Rudolf KD, Partecke BD. Long-term results following denervation of the wrist in patients with stages II and III SLAC/SNAC wrist. Handchir Mikrochir Plast Chir 2006;38:261–6.
17. Schweizer A, Von Kanel O, Kammer E, et al. Long-term follow-up evaluation of denervation of the wrist. J Hand Surg Am 2006;31:559–64.
18. Van de Pol GJ, Koudstaal MJ, Schuurman AH, et al. Innervation of the wrist joint and surgical perspectives of denervation. J Hand Surg Am 2006;31:28–34.
19. Braga-Silva J, Roman JA, Padoin AV. Wrist denervation for painful conditions of the wrist. J Hand Surg Am 2011;36:961–6.
20. Grafe MW, Kim PD, Rosenwasser MP, et al. Wrist denervation and the anterior interosseous nerve: anatomic considerations. J Hand Surg Am 2005;30:1221–5.
21. Lin DL, Lenhart MK, Farber GL. Anatomy of the anterior interosseous innervation of the pronator quadratus: evaluation of structures at risk in the single dorsal incision wrist denervation technique. J Hand Surg Am 2006;31:904–7.
22. Nagle DN. Evaluation of chronic wrist pain. J Am Acad Orthop Surg 2000;8:45–55.

23. Hofmeister EP, Moran SL, Shin AY. Anterior and posterior interosseous neurectomy for the treatment of chronic dynamic instability of the wrist. Hand (N Y) 2006;1(2):63–70.

24. Berger RA. Partial denervation of the wrist: a new approach. Tech Hand Up Extrem Surg 1998;2: 25–35.

25. Delclaux S, Elia F, Bouvet C. Denervation of the wrist with two surgical incisions. Is it effective? A review of 33 patients with an average of 41 months' follow-up. Hand Surg Rehabil 2017; 36(4):281–5.

26. Vanden Berge DJ, Kusnezov NA, Rubin S. Outcomes following isolated posterior interosseous nerve neurectomy: a systematic review. Hand (N Y) 2017;12(6):535–40.

27. Strauch RJ. Denervation of the wrist joint for chronic pain. In: Slutsky DJ, editor. Principles and practice of wrist surgery. 1st edition. Philadelphia: Saunders Elsevier; 2010. p. 624–31.

28. Fuchsberger T, Boesch CE, Tonagel F3. Patient-rated long-term results after complete denervation of the wrist. J Plast Reconstr Aesthet Surg 2018; 71(1):57–61.

29. O'Shaughnessy MA, Wagner ER, Berger RA. Buying time: long-term results of wrist denervation and time to repeat surgery. Hand (N Y) 2018. https:// doi.org/10.1177/1558944718760031.

30. Sgromolo NM, Cho MS, Gower JT2. Partial wrist denervation for idiopathic dorsal wrist pain in an active duty military population. J Hand Surg Am 2018;43(12):1108–12.

31. Gay A, Harbst K, Hansen DK, et al. Effect of partial wrist denervation on wrist kinesthesia: wrist denervation does not impair proprioception. J Hand Surg Am 2011;36(11):1774–9.

32. Tuffaha SH, Quan A, Hashemi S, et al. Selective thumb carpometacarpal joint denervation for painful arthritis: clinical outcomes and cadaveric study. J Hand Surg Am 2019;44(1):64.e1-8.

Subungual Melanoma

Travis W. Littleton, MD[a],*, Peter M. Murray, MD[b,c], Mark E. Baratz, MD[a,1]

KEYWORDS

- Subungual melanoma • Longitudinal melanonychia • Nail matrix • Hutchinson sign • Periungual
- Malignant melanoma • Melanocytes

KEY POINTS

- Subungual melanoma is a rare form of melanoma that presents a unique set of challenges largely based on the complex anatomy of the nail unit.
- A nail-specific "ABCDEF" guide has been developed and can be very useful in the evaluation of longitudinal melanonychia.
- Practitioners must have a high clinical suspicion in the evaluation of any patient with longitudinal melanonychia.
- One of the most consistent findings in early subungual melanoma is periungual pigmentation of the posterior nail fold.
- Biopsy of the nail unit should be performed by a surgeon with an in-depth understanding of the pathoanatomy of the nail matrix and of subungual melanoma.

INTRODUCTION

Subungual melanoma is an uncommon variant of melanoma that arises from the nail matrix and commonly affects other areas of the nail unit.

Definition: Longitudinal melanonychia is defined as a pigmented, often brown or black, streaking of the nail bed (**Fig. 1**).

Melanonychia is a condition caused by hyperplasia or activation of melanocytes. This can be seen in subungual hematoma, bacterial infection, onychomycosis nigricans, human immunodeficiency virus, pigmentation disorders, metabolic deficiencies such as B12 or folate, endocrine disorders, secondary effects of drugs or radiation, and benign masses. However, this also can be the first sign of a subungual malignant melanoma and one must have a high index of suspicion.[1]

Melanonychia is a presenting feature in approximately 70% of subungual melanomas.[2–4] In addition, many people with subungual melanoma report a history of trauma. In this setting, it is appropriate to consider both subungual hematoma and melanoma as possible reasons for the appearance of longitudinal melanonychia.[1] Subungual melanoma is commonly mistaken as an infection. In cases of presumed infection with nail pigmentation, it may be appropriate to obtain a biopsy if the condition fails to respond to treatment after several months.[1] Subungual melanoma should be considered in the differential in any patient with longitudinal melanonychia (**Fig. 1**).

Longitudinal melanonychia originates from the germinal matrix and affects the nail plate preferentially based on whether it comes from the proximal or distal nail matrix. The proximal nail matrix affects the superficial nail plate, whereas the distal nail matrix affects the deep nail plate. This information can be useful and

Disclosure Statement: T.W. Littleton and P.M. Murray have nothing to disclose. M.E. Baratz: Integra Royalties and Speakers Bureau, Elsevier Royalties, RJOS Board Member/Committee Appointment for a Society.
[a] Department of Orthopaedic Surgery, University of Pittsburgh Medical Center, Pittsburgh, PA 15237, USA;
[b] Department of Orthopedic Surgery, Mayo Clinic, 4500 San Pablo Road South #378, Jacksonville, FL 32224, USA; [c] Neurosurgery, Mayo Clinic, 4500 San Pablo Road South #378, Jacksonville, FL 32224, USA
[1]Present address: UPMC South Hills, 1300 Oxford Drive, Suite 1200, Bethel Park, PA 15102.
* Corresponding author. 3333 Forbes Avenue, Apartment 1216, Pittsburgh, PA 15213.
E-mail address: littletontw@upmc.edu

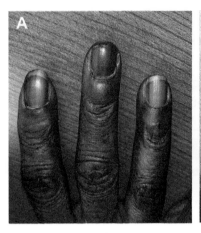
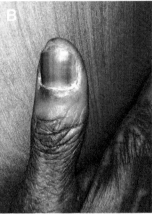

Fig. 1. (*A*, *B*) Benign longitudinal melanonychia. (*Courtesy of* M. Baratz, MD, Pittsburgh, PA.)

obtained by either dermoscopy or a nail clipping stained with Fontana-Masson evaluated by a pathologist.[5]

Definition: Dermoscopy refers to evaluation of the nail and adjacent skin using a dermatoscope that uses magnification and nonpolarized light to improve visualization (**Fig. 2**).

Subungual melanoma originates in the nail matrix and often first appears with longitudinal melanonychia. The typical mode of spread is from the nail matrix directly to the adjacent nail plate and across the nail bed and to the hyponychium and nail folds.[6] This is the explanation for the Hutchinson sign that can be seen in the posterior nail fold, lateral nail fold, and even on the tip of the finger.[7]

Definition: Hutchinson sign is an extension of brown or black pigmentation in the adjacent periungual skin (**Fig. 3**).

The severity progression of melanoma includes benign nevus, melanoma in situ via radial growth, invasive melanoma via vertical growth, and ultimately metastatic melanoma. Increasingly poor prognosis accompanies each advancing stage.[8]

Progression of melanoma:

Benign nevus → melanoma in situ → invasive melanoma → metastatic melanoma

radial growth → vertical growth → lymphatic

The distant spread of subungual melanoma is through the lymphatic system and up to

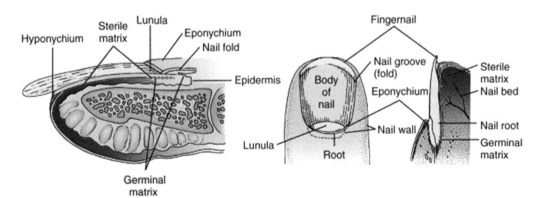

Fig. 2. Nail unit. (*From* Lammers RL, Scrimshaw LE. Methods of wound closure. In: Roberts JR, Custalow CB, Thomsen TW, editors. Roberts and Hedges' clinical procedures in emergency medicine and acute care, 7th edition. Philadelphia: Elsevier; 2019; with permission.)

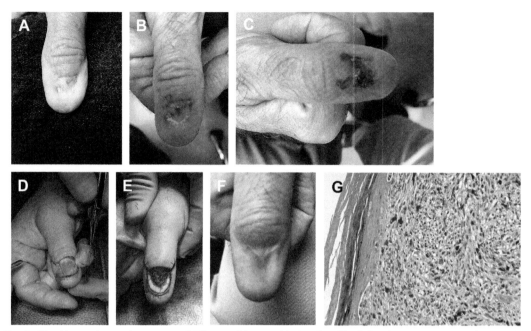

Fig. 3. Hutchinson sign and treatment. A 70-year-old man with thumb nailbed discoloration stemming from a table saw injury 7 years prior leading to dermatology punch biopsy with uncertain pathology. Three years later, the patient presented with persistent nail deformity and discoloration. (A–C) Appearance of thumb 8, 12, and 24 months following a second biopsy showing nuclear atypia (2/mm²) and positive immunostain melatonin A suspicious for malignant melanoma. Note the progression of the Hutchinson sign. Cosmetic deformity resulted in the patient desiring tumor excision and thumb length preservation. (D–F) Composite nail bed marginal excisional biopsy, partial hypothenar skin grafting, and final appearance with residual secondary wound healing. (G) Hematoxylin-eosin stain consistent with superficial spreading melanoma without lymphatic or vascular invasion (H&E, original magnification ×200). (*Courtesy of* J. Calandruccio, MD, Memphis, TN.)

one-quarter of patients can present with lymph node or distant metastasis at presentation.[9]

INCIDENCE AND DEMOGRAPHICS

The incidence of subungual melanoma is equal among all races.[10] However, subungual melanoma accounts for approximately 1% to 3% of cutaneous melanomas in White, but a much higher percentage, 8% to 33% of non-White.[11] The prevalence is much higher in Japanese and in Afro-Caribbean populations, 23% and 25% respectively.[9] Subungual melanomas most commonly occur between the ages of 50 and 70, and have an equal incidence in both men and women. These lesions commonly present with longitudinal melanonychia, nail splitting, or nail bed bleeding and have a predilection for the thumb or index finger.[11]

The incidence of longitudinal melanonychia is much higher in the Japanese population at large (10%), but many of these cases are benign.[10] There is a rare subungual subtype of acral lentiginous melanoma that accounts for fewer than 1% of melanomas across the entire population, but may be as much as 75% of cases in the non-White population.

Definition: Acral lentiginous melanoma is a specific type of melanoma that occurs in the extremities on the palms, soles of the feet, or under the nails.

This acral lentiginous melanoma has an increased mortality and may be secondary to these pigmented lesions being in less noticeable areas and more difficult to distinguish in darker skinned individuals.[12] Byrd and colleagues[13] reported a significantly decreased 5-year survival rate in African American individuals, (59%) as compared with an 85% 5-year survival in White.

INITIAL EVALUATION
History
Obtain a detailed history when evaluating for any presumed cutaneous malignancy in the upper extremity. Focus on both the recent and remote changes in size, appearance, and color of the lesion. Melanomas often extend past the visible margin of the lesion. This is particularly important when evaluating

subungual melanomas and their vertical margins because there is very little subcutaneous tissue between the skin and the deeper structures: dermis and bone. Melanoma constitutes a very small percentage of skin cancers, but accounts for more than 75% of all deaths from skin cancers.[8] Subungual melanoma carries an especially poor prognosis. In a study out of the United Kingdom, Miranda and colleagues[14] reported a disproportionately poor prognosis with a 5-year survival rate of 25% to 51%.

In addition, many people with subungual melanoma report a history of trauma, so one should not immediately dismiss longitudinal melanonychia as simply being a hematoma. Nail trauma has been theoreticized as a cause of subungual melanoma; this has not proven to be true, but trauma may draw attention to previously unrecognized melanoma.

CLINICAL EVALUATION

A nail-specific "ABCDEF" guide was developed to examine risk factors associated with subungual melanoma (**Fig. 4**), originally presented by Levit and colleagues[15] in 2000.

These factors are designed to be used in combination and not in isolation, as the more positive findings in each case increase the risk of the lesion being malignant:

- "A" stands for Age.
  - The highest incidence is in individuals 50 to 70 years old.
  - "A" can also be used for races with increased incidence: African American, Native American, and Asian.
- "B" stands for Band width.
  - Irregular Borders.
  - "B" also stands for Brown or Black color of the pigmented lesion.

- "C" stands for Changes in the appearance of the lesion.
- "D" refers to the Digit involved.
  - Subungual melanoma primarily affects a single digit with the thumb and index finger being the most common.
- "E" represents Extension of the lesion into the surrounding skin.
  - Hutchinson sign.
- "F" stands for Family or personal history.[15]

This is not all encompassing in the clinical evaluation of a pigmented lesion of the nail. Therefore, any lesion with concerning history or appearance should undergo a biopsy regardless of the number of positive criteria.

A high index of suspicion is helpful when evaluating melanonychia.[11] Brown discoloration is characteristic of melanocytic hyperplasia, and in association with an irregular appearance may be a melanoma. The lesion width or diameter is important, as a width >3 to 6 mm correlates with at increased risk of malignancy.[8] In addition, a band that is wider proximally than distally is often representative of a rapidly growing melanoma. Associated nail fold pigmentation, known as Hutchinson sign, is due to radial growth of the neoplasm and is pathognomonic of subungual melanoma.[5]

DERMOSCOPY

Dermoscopic evaluation can be a very helpful adjunct in distinguishing between subungual melanoma and benign melanocytic pigmented lesions. Dermoscopy is a noninvasive procedure performed by using a dermatoscope with the use of magnification, illumination, and a gel medium to evaluate the areas of pigmentation and characteristics of the underlying lesion. A dermatoscope allows for more microscopic

ABCDEF		
A	Age (5–7th decade)	Race: African American, Native American, Asian at increased risk
B	Nail Band: Breadth >3mm or irregular Borders	Brown to Black discoloration of the pigmented lesion
C	Change	
D	Digit involved (most commonly thumb and index finger) single Digit > multiple digits.	
E	Extension of pigment into the nail fold (Hutchinson sign)	
F	Family or personal history	

Fig. 4. "ABCDEF" rule. (*From* Levit EK, Kagen MH, Scher RK, et al. The ABC rule for clinical detection of subungual melanoma. J Am Acad Dermatol 2000;42(2 Pt 1):269–74; with permission.)

visualization of subsurface structures that are not visible to the naked eye. Some characteristics suggestive of melanoma include irregular bands of brown or black pigmentation, lines that are not parallel, blurred ill-defined borders, width >3 mm, nail dystrophy, nail fold ulceration, and Hutchinson sign. Dermoscopy is very helpful in distinguishing between subungual melanoma and benign melanocytic pigmented lesions.[11] Dermoscopy also can be used to aid in defining periungual skin involvement. However, biopsy of any pigmented area remains the gold standard for establishing a diagnosis of subungual melanoma.

It is important to biopsy any portion of the finger that shows any signs of pigmentation. Hoashi and colleagues[6] reported a case of subungual melanoma with subtle clinical findings and found atypical melanocytes only in the nail matrix and surrounding periungual skin. They concluded that malignant atypical melanocytes occur more commonly in the nail matrix, the nail folds, and hyponychium rather than in the nail bed itself. This again emphasizes the value to biopsy any area of abnormal pigmentation.

BIOPSY

Subungual melanomas originate in the nail matrix and spread out to the adjacent nail bed. From here, the lesion can invade the periungual skin via radial growth. It also can invade the dermis via vertical growth and eventually invade the underlying bone.[6] Biopsy is requisite for the diagnosis of subungual melanoma. However, the diagnosis can still be missed or be inconclusive on initial biopsy. Both shave and punch biopsies have been described for a pigmented lesion of the nail plate, but these methods often fail to determine the actual depth of tumor invasion. We recommend longitudinal full-thickness excisional biopsies of the pigmented area(s), including the nail folds or fingertip skin. Suspicious lesions require a biopsy, ideally performed under local anesthesia after atraumatic nail plate removal. The specimen should be full-thickness and longitudinally oriented and excise only the entire lesion if nail bed approximation is possible pending definitive histologic diagnosis to prevent nail plate deformities should the process be benign.

INDICATIONS FOR BIOPSY

- Longitudinal melanonychia in a single digit, especially the thumb or index

- Any change in the appearance of longitudinal melanonychia
- Proximal width greater than distal width of melanonychia
- Any pigmented lesion associated with infection that does not respond to treatment
- Relative indication: band width >3 mm. Absolute indication: band width >6 mm
- Irregular, jagged, or indistinct borders of melanonychia
- History of melanoma: personal or family
- Nail bleeding, dystrophy, or ulceration
- Hutchinson sign

Miranda and colleagues[14] reported a case with discoloration of the nail, with less pigmented skin adjacent to the nail. The initial biopsy of the sterile and germinal nail matrix failed to show evidence of malignancy. However, due to the high clinical suspicion, a second biopsy was performed and the histopathology from the less deeply pigmented skin lesion showed an increase in abnormal melanocytes. This was consistent with a diagnosis of acral lentiginous melanoma in situ and the patient was treated with an amputation through the middle phalanx, demonstrating the importance of biopsying all potentially involved areas.

Even with meticulous technique, the thickness of the lesion is often underestimated. Reilly and colleagues[16] retrospectively reviewed 54 patients with subungual melanomas and found that their initial biopsy was inaccurate in 45% of patients because the final thickness was greater than the thickness found at initial biopsy. This is believed to be because the interface between layers is often indistinct and can be distorted secondary to tumor invasion.

BIOPSY TECHNIQUE

- The patient should be advised on the risk of nail dystrophy following biopsy.[17]
- Most biopsies can be safely performed under local anesthesia. A digital tourniquet is often used after gravity exsanguination of the extremity to help make sure the appropriate pigmented area is sampled. Alternately, epinephrine may be used with the local anesthesia and a tourniquet avoided.
- The nail plate is carefully elevated off of the underlying nail bed. Removal of the nail plate can be performed using a number of instruments, such as a Freer elevator, iris scissors, or even a 15-blade

scalpel. Elevation of the proximal nail fold is also sometimes required. A hemostat is then used to grasp the distal extent of the nail plate and atraumatically rock back and forth to detach the nail plate.

- Two oblique incisions in the corners of the eponychial fold allow better visualization of the germinal matrix more proximally.
- Under ×2.5 to ×3.5 loupe magnification define the extent of the entire lesion including any area of abnormal pigmentation, ulceration, or dystrophy of the nail bed or adjacent skin and nail folds.
- The biopsy should be performed using a fresh 15-blade, obtaining a biopsy specimen of the abnormal nail bed and germinal matrix down to the periosteum. The biopsy must also include any periungual skin involvement.
- This biopsy site may be closed primarily using a side-to-side closure with absorbable suture. The eponychial folds should be repaired in a similar fashion.
- A sterile nonadherent dressing is placed over the biopsy site and splinting of the nail can be performed with an inert material such as a piece of aluminum foil from a suture packet or a section of a disposable bowl from the surgical pack. This can be temporarily sutured in place to prevent scarring/adherence of the eponychial fold to the underling nail bed.

PATHOLOGY

Kerl and colleagues[18] described histologic criteria in the cornified layer of the epidermis to differentiate a melanocytic nevus from a malignant melanoma in the nail bed. Some of their keys to distinguish the difference include the following:

- Numerous melanocytes and melanin granules
- Melanin diffusely distributed
- Atypical melanocytes (pleomorphism, cellular atypia, mitotic figures) (see Fig. 3G)

These are subtle findings to help aid in the diagnosis of malignant melanoma, as melanocytes can be found even in the cornified layer of benign melanocytic nevi.[18]

Histopathology is required for diagnosis of subungual melanoma and certain stains such as Fontana-Masson aid in the diagnosis. Immunostains (MART-1, Melan-A, S-100, HMB-45, and NKI/C3 protein markers) also may aid in the diagnosis.[19,20] A positive MART-1 or HMB45 and S-100 protein with negative cytokeratin confirms the diagnosis of melanoma.[15] More recent literature has shown the superiority of MART-1 over HMB45 as a more sensitive and easier to interpret stain. Terushkin and colleagues[20] reported no local recurrence in 34 patients with the use of Mohs surgery after switching to MART-1 staining from HMB45.

WIDE SURGICAL EXCISION

Due to the intimate relationship of the nail matrix, nail bed, and underlying bone, the Breslow depth criteria is less helpful. Melanoma in situ is defined as a tumor that does not extend the entire depth of the nail matrix. Some surgeons have recommended Mohs surgery for melanoma in situ. This, however, has been mostly been described in case reports and in one study by Brodland[21] looking at 14 patients treated with Mohs surgery with variable results.[22] However, one study by Terushkin and colleagues[20] showed great results with treatment of subungual melanoma with Mohs surgery. They reported local recurrence-free survival of 92% and 83% at 5 and 10 years. Interestingly, 95% of individuals with primary disease were able to avoid amputation. They also noted improved results with the use of MART-1 staining over HMB45.[20]

More commonly it is recommended that subungual melanomas be managed with wide surgical excision or amputation with or without sentinel node biopsy. Historically, amputations have been through the phalanx proximal to the lesion. More recently, some investigators have proposed amputations through the most distal uninvolved interphalangeal (IP) joint, that is, the IP joint in the thumb.[8]

Ishihara and colleagues[10] proposed the term "ungual" malignant melanoma in 1993 as opposed to subungual because these tumors are believed to originate from the nail matrix itself. They also state that ungual melanoma in situ has "no risk for developing metastasis" and subsequently recommend wide resection and not amputation.

However, in a series of 13 cases of melanoma in situ treated with wide local excision, there were 4 recurrences. Two were benign lesions, but the other 2 had recurrence with an invasive melanoma. The 2 recurrent malignancies were treated by thumb IP joint disarticulation. Unfortunately, both of these patients required a third operation and more proximal amputation for positive margins.[26] Some, therefore, recommend primary interphalangeal joint disarticulation for melanoma in situ of the thumb. This has been proposed by both Quinn[23] and O'Leary[24] with reports of no differences in survival or recurrence.[22]

Sureda and colleagues[12] reported on wide local excision and full-thickness skin grafting with no recurrence at an average follow-up of 45 months. This was a series of 7 patients, all with melanoma in situ or minimally invasive subungual melanoma.

Distal IP joint disarticulation carries no increased risk of recurrence compared with more proximal amputation levels. Mannava and colleagues[5] recommended proximal IP joint disarticulation in involved fingers or through the proximal phalanx of the thumb for invasive melanomas as long as clear margins are obtained.

Nguyen and colleagues[3] reported on a series of 124 cases at the Mayo Clinic over a 96-year period looking at the surgical management of subungual melanoma with a mean length of 2.2 years between symptom onset and diagnosis. This series looked at subungual melanoma in both the upper and lower extremities with 79 occurring in the hand. The average Breslow depth was 3.1 mm and these patients were treated with amputation at a number of different levels. They found an overall poor prognosis with a 59% disease-specific survival rates at 5 years. Despite a poor prognosis, level of resection was not significantly associated with survival or disease progression as long as histologically free margins were obtained intraoperatively. They recommended distal IP joint amputations in the fingers and IP joint amputations of the thumb. However, they also discuss the importance of maintaining length in the thumb and considering more length-sparing amputations for thumb subungual melanoma.

One option for treatment of thumb subungual melanoma is resection of the thumb nail and tissue down to bone and coverage with a superthin free superficial circumflex iliac artery perforator (SCIP) flap. This was reported by Lee and colleagues[2] in a study of 41 patients with primary subungual melanoma less than or equal to 2 mm in thickness treated with functional surgical excision and an SCIP flap. The average SCIP flap was inset with an average thickness of 1.5 to 4.0 mm at inset. They found that this thin free flap was adequate to cover exposed bone of the distal phalanx with low complication rates, rapid wound healing, and minimal morbidity. Most patients had complete wound healing by 3 weeks, and there was only 1

complete flap failure. There was a low rate of recurrence in the study by Lee and colleagues,[2] with recurrence of only 2 (4.9%) of 41 patients. The average time to recurrence was 2 years and 7 months. All of these patients had early melanoma with a lesion depth <2 mm, which is significantly less than other studies with reported average depths of 4 to 5 mm.[2] Coverage after wide local excision can also be provided with a full-thickness skin graft. This has been reported on by Sureda and others[12] with good cosmetic and functional results. Full-thickness skin grafting is a simpler and less technically demanding option for coverage after wide local excision of a subungual melanoma and can be applied directly to the exposed distal phalanx. Finally, healing by secondary intention is acceptable as well (see **Fig. 3F**).

The authors do not believe there is enough evidence to routinely recommend digit preservation procedures for subungual malignant melanoma for more advanced lesions such as invasive or recurrent disease. Both Finley[25] and O'Leary[24] reported on their experiences with distal interphalangeal joint disarticulations and reported no recurrences.[22] For such lesions we recommend amputation at the level of the most distal unaffected joint.

MARGINS

Tumor-free resection margins vary according to various sources. Unfortunately, there is insufficient evidence to determine the appropriate tumor depth and width of resection to eliminate local disease persistence or recurrence. The recommendations for management of melanomas in general include the following:

1. National Institute for Health and Care Excellence: 0.5 cm for stage 0, 1 cm for stage I, and >2 cm in stage II.
2. American Academy of Dermatology: 0.5 to 1.0 cm for in situ tumors, 1 cm for tumors up to 1 cm depth, 1 to 2 cm for tumors 1 to 2 cm, and a minimum resection of 2 mm for tumors >2 cm invasion.[26]
3. Martin and colleagues[22]: Invasive melanoma <1 mm thickness requires 1-cm margin. Lesions 1 to 2 mm in depth require 1- to 2-cm margins. Lesions 2 to 4 mm in depth require 1- to 3-cm margins. Large lesions >4 mm in thickness require 3-cm margins.
4. O'Connor and Dzwierzynski[1]: Melanoma in situ: 2- to 5-mm margin. Invasive melanoma <1 mm thickness requires 1-cm margin.

Invasive melanoma >1 mm thickness requires a 2-cm margin.[1]

However, the preceding recommendations for melanomas elsewhere cannot apply to subungual melanomas due to the unique and compact nailbed anatomy.

ROLE FOR LYMPH NODE BIOPSY

Subungual melanoma may warrant clinical evaluation of lymph node involvement for staging purposes; this includes melanoma in situ and invasive melanoma. However, 2 large randomized controlled trials showed no additional benefit to elective lymph node dissection and now sentinel lymph node biopsy is more commonly recommended and performed.[22] Sentinel lymph node biopsy studies have shown that approximately 15% of subungual melanomas have metastasized at diagnosis.[5] Other studies have estimated that up to one-quarter of patients can present with lymph node or distant metastasis at presentation.[9] In a randomized controlled trial by Martin and colleagues,[22] there was an increased survival at 5 years with sentinel lymph node biopsy in conjunction with wide local excision. Sentinel lymph node biopsy is recommended in any lesion >1 mm thickness or in lesions <1 mm but with a mitosis rate greater than $1/mm^2$ as these characteristics are predictive of more aggressive lesions. Any positive sentinel lymph node biopsy should be further evaluated with a regional lymph node dissection. In a study by Reilly and colleagues,[16] sentinel lymph node biopsy was performed in 36 patients with subungual melanoma. Positive sentinel lymph node biopsy was found in 11 of 36 patients; however, this was also accompanied by a false-negative rate of 35%.

One of the proposed reasons for the poor prognosis with subungual melanoma is the concern for metastasis at diagnosis. Therefore, there may be a role for sentinel lymph node biopsy despite no level 1 evidence.[27] Clinical suspicion should still be high even with a negative sentinel lymph node biopsy due to the high false-negative rates in the literature.[16]

SPECIAL CIRCUMSTANCES

Another uncommon cause of a pigmented lesion in or around the nail is tumoral melanosis. Tumoral melanosis is a rare form of a regressed melanoma. Most melanoma cells are replaced with melanophages, which are melanin-laden macrophages. High clinical suspicion and dermoscopy is the key to an accurate diagnosis.

One must look for a parallel ridge pattern of residual melanoma cells often at the distal edge of the tumor. The recommended treatment of tumoral melanosis is amputation and sentinel node biopsy.[28]

COMPLICATIONS AND MANAGEMENT

Early detection and treatment of subungual melanoma should minimize the risk of metastasis and subsequently improve survival associated with subungual melanoma. Cure of melanoma in situ and early-stage disease is possible; therefore, our goal as treating physicians should be prevention by earlier detection. Gosselink and colleagues[19] estimated that 85% of subungual melanomas are initially misdiagnosed. Numerous case reports show a delay in diagnosis resulting in higher mortality (**Fig. 5**).

POSTOPERATIVE CARE

Ilyas and colleagues[17] recommend regular dermatology follow-up for any patient with a subungual melanoma. Mannava and colleagues[5] recommend referral to medical oncology and advanced imaging in the form of computed tomography (CT) and/or MRI of brain, chest, abdomen, and pelvis versus a whole-body PET-CT in any stage III or IV melanoma (metastatic melanoma). Management of stage IV melanoma may also include chemotherapy, radiation, immunotherapy, or possibly molecularly targeted therapy. BRAF inhibition is a molecular targeted therapy with promising results in select subsets of patients. There are emerging data on the role of molecular studies to help diagnose and detect recurrence. Two more recent

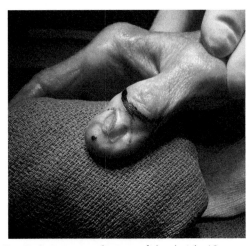

Fig. 5. Recurrent melanoma of the thumb. (*Courtesy of* P. Murray, MD, Jacksonville, FL.)

molecular studies include the BRAF and KIT, which can aid in adjuvant treatment options.[16]

The current recommendations for chemotherapy are largely left to the medical and/or surgical oncologist, but should be considered in stage III and IV subungual melanoma.

OUTCOMES

Melanoma makes up less than 5% of skin cancers, but accounts for greater than 75% of all deaths from skin cancers. Subungual melanoma has a very poor prognosis and prognosis is associated with tumor depth and staging.[8] In a report published in 1993 from Japan, the investigators reported a 3.1-year average survival in patients diagnosed with fingernail melanoma. Unfortunately, over the past 25 years, not much progress has been made in survival improvement despite increased awareness of these lesions.[10]

One study published 5-year and 10-year survival rates of subungual melanoma of 30% and 13%, respectively.[11] Another reported a wide range of 5-year survival of subungual melanoma from 16% to 87%. Survival is best linked to depth of invasion, with Breslow thickness being the most predicative finding.

SUMMARY

"If a malignant process cannot be clearly ruled out, histopathologic examination of the nail bed and the germinal matrix should be done"—Braun and Gerber.[29] This conclusion highlights the importance of pathologic evaluation of any pigmented lesion of the nail unit.[29] The real issue in treatment of subungual melanoma is that there are no randomized or prospective studies comparing marginal versus wide excision, including amputation level. The low incidence of subungual melanoma and the heterogeneity of the lesions makes definitive treatment difficult to determine.[22]

Izumi and colleagues[7] looked at 50 cases of subungual melanoma and divided them into 4 groups based on clinical stage, and then carefully examined their histologic appearances. Based on these findings, the investigators were able to make some correlations and findings that help distinguish a malignant process. This study came up with 3 pathologic clues to help diagnose early-stage subungual melanoma:

- First is "skip lesions" (proliferation of the tumor cells is more prominent in the hyponychium than in the nail bed or nail matrix).

- Second, histologic confirmation of a Hutchinson sign.
  - The importance of these first 2 histologic findings is that they are not seen in benign conditions and, therefore, are essentially diagnostic of subungual melanoma.
- Third, epithelial thickening and/or compact arrangement of elongated basal cells.

These findings can be seen even before the ability to detect mitoses. In this study, mitoses were not seen until the progressive stage, but these other clues were found in the earlier stages. The most consistent finding in early-stage subungual melanoma was histologic periungual pigmentation in the posterior nail fold in all 19 patients in the early stage.[7]

In conclusion, malignancy should be considered in any patient with a longitudinal melanonychia, and a biopsy performed routinely in suspicious lesions. The "ABCDEF" guide can be a useful tool to aid in screening any lesion of the nail bed. We recommend that biopsies of the nail unit be performed by a surgeon with an understanding of the pathoanatomy of subungual melanoma and a consultation for adjunct therapy be determined with an appropriate oncologist.

REFERENCES

1. O'Connor EA, Dzwierzynski W. Longitudinal melonychia: clinical evaluation and biopsy technique [review]. J Hand Surg Am 2011;36(11):1852–4.
2. Lee KT, Park BY, Kim EJ, et al. Superthin SCIP flap for reconstruction of subungual melanoma: aesthetic functional surgery. Plast Reconstr Surg 2017;140(6):1278–89.
3. Nguyen JT, Bakri K, Nguyen EC, et al. Surgical management of subungual melanoma: mayo clinic experience of 124 cases. Ann Plast Surg 2013;71(4):346–54.
4. Glat PM, Spector JA, Roses DF, et al. The management of pigmented lesions of the nail bed. Ann Plast Surg 1996;37(2):125–34.
5. Mannava KA, Mannava S, Koman LA, et al. Longitudinal melanonychia: detection and management of nail melanoma [review]. Hand Surg 2013;18(1):133–9.
6. Hoashi T, Funasaka Y, Shirakawa N, et al. Case of subungual malignant melanoma showing the subtle clinical features and unexpected typical histopathological findings of melanoma in situ. J Dermatol 2016;43(11):1361–2.
7. Izumi M, Ohara K, Hoashi T, et al. Subungual melanoma: histological examination of 50 cases from early stage to bone invasion. J Dermatol 2008; 35(11):695–703.

8. English C, Hammert WC. Cutaneous malignancies of the upper extremity [review]. J Hand Surg Am 2012;37(2):367–77.

9. Amin K, Edmonds K, Fleming A, et al. Subungual malignant melanoma–re-learning the lesson. BMJ Case Rep 2011. https://doi.org/10.1136/bcr.10.2010.3422.

10. Ishihara Y, Matsumoto K, Kawachi S, et al. Detection of early lesions of "ungual" malignant melanoma. Int J Dermatol 1993;32(1):44–7.

11. Dunphy L, Morhij R, Verma Y, et al. Missed opportunity to diagnose subungual melanoma: potential pitfalls! BMJ Case Rep 2017. https://doi.org/10.1136/bcr-2016-218785.

12. Sureda N, Phan A, Poulalhon N, et al. Conservative surgical management of subungual (matrix derived) melanoma: report of seven cases and literature review [review]. Br J Dermatol 2011;165(4):852–8.

13. Stubblefield J, Kelly B. Melanoma in non-Caucasian populations [review]. Surg Clin North Am 2014; 94(5):1115–26, ix.

14. Miranda BH, Haughton DN, Fahmy FS. Subungual melanoma: an important tip. J Plast Reconstr Aesthet Surg 2012;65(10):1422–4.

15. Levit EK, Kagen MH, Scher RK, et al. The ABC rule for clinical detection of subungual melanoma [review]. J Am Acad Dermatol 2000;42(2 Pt 1): 269–74.

16. Reilly DJ, Aksakal G, Gilmour RF, et al. Subungual melanoma: management in the modern era. J Plast Reconstr Aesthet Surg 2017;70(12):1746–52.

17. Ilyas EN, Leinberry CF, Ilyas AM. Skin cancers of the hand and upper extremity [review]. J Hand Surg Am 2012;37(1):171–8.

18. Kerl H, Trau H, Ackerman AB. Differentiation of melanocytic nevi from malignant melanomas in palms, soles, and nail beds solely by signs in the cornified layer of the epidermis. Am J Dermatopathol 1984;6(Suppl):159–60.

19. Gosselink CP, Sindone JL, Meadows BJ, et al. Amelanotic subungual melanoma: a case report. J Foot Ankle Surg 2009;48(2):220–4.

20. Terushkin V, Brodland DG, Sharon DJ, et al. Digit-sparing Mohs surgery for melanoma [review]. Dermatol Surg 2016;42(1):83–93.

21. Brodland DG. The treatment of nail apparatus melanoma with Mohs micrographic surgery. Dermatol Surg 2001;27:269–73.

22. Martin DE, English JC, Goitz RJ. Subungual malignant melanoma [review]. J Hand Surg Am 2011; 36(4):704–7.

23. Quinn MJ, Thompson JE, Crotty K, et al. Subungual melanoma of the hand. J Hand Surg 1996;21A: 506–11.

24. O'Leary JA, Berend KR, Johnson JL, et al. Subungual melanoma. A review of 93 cases with identification of prognostic variables. Clin Orthop Relat Res 2000;378:206–12.

25. Finley RK III, Driscoll DL, Blumenson LE, et al. Subungual melanoma: An eighteen-year review. Surgery 1994;116:96–100.

26. Sinno S, Wilson S, Billig J, et al. Primary melanoma of the hand: an algorithmic approach to surgical management. J Plast Surg Hand Surg 2015;49(6): 339–45.

27. Chakera AH, Quinn MJ, Lo S, et al. Subungual melanoma of the hand. Ann Surg Oncol 2018. https://doi.org/10.1245/s10434-018-07094-w.

28. Kato K, Namiki T, Nojima K, et al. Case of subungual tumoral melanosis: the detection of melanoma cells and dermoscopic features. J Dermatol 2018;45(6):e161–2.

29. Braun S, Gerber P. Subungual malignant melanoma. CMAJ 2015;187(12):909.

Fracture Fixation Using Shape-Memory (Ninitol) Staples

John C. Wu, MD[a,*], Andrew Mills, MD[b],
Kevin D. Grant, MD[b], Patrick J. Wiater, MD[b]

KEYWORDS

- Ninitol • Shape memory • Implants • Staples • Fracture fixation

KEY POINTS

- Shape-memory alloy (SMA) staples have been used successfully for osteotomies, arthrodesis, and fracture fixation, especially in small bones.
- SMA staples have inherent compressive properties that create a stable fracture environment that promotes primary bone healing, most effective for transverse fracture patterns.
- Current literature evaluating the indications for staple use, their biomechanical properties, comparison to alternative implants, and functional outcomes is limited.
- Understanding where SMA staple compression can be optimized and using proper indications are important factors for achieving consistent widespread success and minimizing failures.
- SMA staples are not a substitute for lag screw fixation or traditional plate and screw constructs, but are simply another tool that can be used for effective fracture fixation.

INTRODUCTION

Nitinol is a shape memory alloy (SMA) composed of nickel and titanium. The use of nitinol is ubiquitous in endovascular stents and has proven both safe and effective. The alloy is not new to orthopedic fracture surgery, as there have been descriptions of usage dating back to the 1980's. However there has been a resurgence in the use of nitinol orthopaedic implants primarily in foot and ankle as well as hand surgery. Currently, SMA staples are used as stand-alone implants for interfragmentary compression across osteotomies, arthrodeses, as well as for fracture fixation. Recent reports of orthopaedic use of staple fixation have included first metatarsophalangeal joint arthrodesis,[1] scaphoid fractures,[2] intercarpal fusion,[3] and patellar fractures.[4] They also have been used for ligament fixation, facial fractures and reconstructions, and spinal procedures.[5] Successful growth modulation with SMA staples has been reported in animal models.[6]

HISTORY OF SHAPE-MEMORY ALLOY STAPLE FIXATION

NITINOL is an acronym derived from the alloy's elemental composition as well as its place of discovery: Nickel titanium–Naval Ordinance Laboratory. The alloy was discovered in 1959 by William J Buehler and Frederick Wang who were given the task of developing a better alloy for the U.S. Navy Polaris re-entry vehicle.[7,8] When they mixed nickel and titanium in roughly equal anatomic percentages, they discovered an alloy that behaved completely dissimilar to other known alloys. It took about 20 years for science to catch up with this discovery and explain its material properties and inner

[a] Department of Orthopaedic Surgery and Biomedical Engineering, University of Tennessee-Campbell Clinic, 1211 Union Avenue, Suite 510, Memphis, TN 38104, USA; [b] Department of Orthopaedic Surgery and Trauma, Beaumont Health, 3535 West 13 Mile Road, Suite 744, Royal Oak, MI 48073, USA
* Corresponding author.
E-mail address: jwu@campbellclinic.com

Orthop Clin N Am 50 (2019) 367–374
https://doi.org/10.1016/j.ocl.2019.02.002

workings. Nitinol has two unique properties that make it attractive for fracture surgery: pseudoelasticity (or super-elasticity) and shape memory.

Pseudoelasticity is an elastic response to an applied stress that is caused by a phase transformation. A pseudoelastic alloy is able to constantly unload stress over high strains to regain its original shape, much like a spring or rubber band. Common orthopedic alloys such as titanium and 316 L stainless steel can tolerate strain of about 0.25% to 0.5% before plastic deformation occurs. Nitinol on the other hand can absorb up to 8% strain before it enters the plastic deformation slope on the stress-strain curve.[9] Therefore, nitinol is 16 to 32 times more elastic than other alloys used in orthopaedic surgery and demonstrates tremendous endurance.[9]

Shape memory is the ability to undergo reversible deformation with changes in temperature. Nitinol can exist in 1 of 2 solid-state phases, martensite and austenite. Below the transition temperature (martensitic phase), nitinol exhibits extremely elastic properties. Somewhat paradoxically, above the transition temperature (austenitic phase), nitinol releases energy causing it to return to a more stable conformation and become more rigid. The ability of nitinol to readily deform at cooler temperature and then recover its original shape and become more rigid upon warming is a unique material property of this alloy.

The transition temperature can be modified by altering the ratio of nickel and titanium. As a result, most SMA nitinol staple implants are manufactured to have a transition temperature just below body temperature. The resting shape of SMA staples is manufactured to have the bridge and tines in the closed position. The implant is then cooled to its martinsitic phase which makes it flexible. The staple is opened without plastically deformation, and then it is loaded onto and retained by the insertion tool and the open, active position. The tines of the staple are perpendicular to the transverse limb of the staple after loading, facilitating insertion. the ambient body temperature releases the potential energy stored in the implant causing it to return to its original, stable configuration causing the tines to close toward the center of implant. When energy stored in the implant is released to the bone, the work performed is continuous interfragmentary compression. The SMA staple will exert continuous compressive forces across the fracture site until the implant has fully returned to the resting shape. This property differentiates SMA staples from conventional staples that lack these compressive properties.[10,11]

CLINICAL USE OF SHAPE-MEMORY ALLOY STAPLES

The popularity of SMA staples has increased in recent years, and currently multiple sizes and configurations exist including various staple widths, lengths of the transverse limb or legs, and the number of legs on each staple. To date, these implants have been marketed and designed for use in the wrist, hand, and foot and currently available staple sizes and geometries are best suited for those anatomic locations. Despite the current popularity of these implants, few studies exist that examine the biomechanical performance of these implants.[12,13] However, a recent biomechanical study demonstrated that nitinol staple lengths that were 2 mm short of the far cortex resulted in the same compression as a bicortical staple, supporting the idea that bicortical placement is not necessary to obtain adequate compression.[14] The same study found that troughing of bone, to minimize implant prominence, did not weaken the biomechanical properties of the construct and that double staple constructs doubled the compressive force and increased bending strength by greater than 90%.

Although the clinical uses of SMA staples are varied and include use as compressive devices for fixation of osteotomies, small bone arthrodesis, and fracture fixation, clinical studies are limited. The current literature describing indications of SMA staple fixation includes metatarsophalangeal joint arthrodesis,[1] scaphoid fractures,[2] and intercarpal fusion,[3] however, the majority of these publications are limited to cadaver or animal models. In 1987, Yang and colleagues[15] reported the earliest clinical review of fracture fixation using nitinol staples, documenting 51 procedures for fractures and arthrodeses, most of which were in the foot and ankle. The study also reported staple use in fractures of the patella, olecranon, wrist, and metacarpal/phalanges. A later study reported outcomes of 158 intra-articular fractures stabilized with nitinol staples.[16] In that study, satisfactory treatment of fractures of the medial and lateral malleoli, tibial plateau, and lateral humeral condyle were also described.

Indications for Staple Fixation

Indications for SMA staple use are still being determined. These implants are useful for generating continuous interfragmentary compression with the goal being primary bone healing. Traditional orthopaedic implants composed of stainless steel or titanium have limited capacity to store or release energy; hence, these alloys can create only static interfragmentary compression from an exogenous energy source (interfragmentary compression screws, compression plate osteosynthesis). Nitinol staples are a useful adjunct for fracture patterns in which traditional techniques for interfragmentary compression are less effective or difficult to employ. These implants are particularly useful for transverse diaphyseal fractures and can be utilized throughout the body including the clavicle, scapula, long bones of the upper and lower extremity, as well as the pelvis and acetabulum. Advantages include improved accuracy and efficiency in translating provisional fracture reductions into definitive fixation constructs, as well as ease and reproducibility of application. The nascent techniques described here are consistent with AO principles-the only difference being the mode of generating interfragmentary compression. Potential contraindications of SMA staple use include severely osteoporotic bone, absent or poor cortical bone quality, and fractures with significant comminution resulting in small-sized fragments.

How nitinol staples fit in with traditional fracture fixation?

Minimax fracture fixation was popularized by the influential Bernhard Weber.[17] Adjunct SMA staple constructs are an extrapolation of his minimax fracture fixation concept: smaller problem focused implants used to do a specific job (provisional reduction, interfragmentary compression) that are then supported by a more robust fracture neutralization construct, such as a plate, medullary based implant, or an external fixation frame.

Shape memory alloy staples are most useful in appendicular skeletal fracture patterns that are not readily amenable to conventional interfragmentary compression techniques such as leg screws, compression plate osteosynthesis, or the usage of an articulated tensioning device or some variation thereof. Compression plate osteosynthesis can be challenging and time consuming to execute correctly and is dependent on a perfect plate contour and on adequate bone stock to generate sufficient friction between the plate and bone.

A transverse fracture plane can be anatomically reduced with orthogonal linear compression clamps, such as a Weber tenaculum. The transition of this provisional fracture reduction into definitive fixation can be done accurately and efficiently with the use of SMA staples. The staple can be located on the bony surface immediately adjacent to the proposed neutralization implant. Once anatomic reduction is obtained, the transverse limb of the staple is measured (bridge size) to adequately span the fracture and any potential nondisplaced comminution such as a butterfly fragment. Some systems have multiple staple sizes from miniature to robust and have a guide for determining the appropriate bridge length. A drill guide is used for accurate placement. The first hole is drilled in the desired location through the far cortex, and a pull-pin is placed through the guide and the hole. Adjustments can be made by rotating the guide with the pull-pin acting as the center of rotation. The second hole is then drilled, which will set the definitive position of the staple. The length of each staple leg is measured using a depth gauge. The longest acceptable length for the legs of the staple should be chosen to allow the SMA staple to compress both the near cortex and far cortex along the length of the limb, providing adequate stability and compression across the entire fracture site.[11,14]

SMA staples are implanted with an inserting device that keeps the bridge and legs in the open activated conformation. The tips of the legs are aligned with the drill holes, and the staple is partially inserted by hand. The inserters have a quick release that disengages the staple, and then the staple is fully inserted with a tamp. In circumstances where impacting the staple is not desired, the staple can by gently seated using a lobster claw clamp between the staple bridge and the far cortex. This is preferable to impacting one leg at a time, which can cause the staple to be inserted off axis. Interfragmentary compression occurs immediately once the insertion device is released and continues until the fracture gap is limited by fracture apposition. Multiple staples can be placed orthogonal about the fracture if it requires compression from various vectors. Double-staple constructs were shown to have better bending stiffness than a single-staple construct, regardless of the plane of the deforming load.[12,14,18]

The Hueter-Volkmann Law states that compressive forces on bone lead to resorption. Resorption at a fracture surface under static compression can potentially lead to destabilization of the construct and loss of interfragmentary compression. With SMA staple constructs, bone resorption or fracture settling will not disrupt the interfragmentary compression so long as the bridge and legs of the staple have not retained the resting or closed position. In our experience, most SMA staples remain in open activated position through bony union indicating that the fracture surfaces are under continuous interfragmentary compression throughout the healing phase.

Efficiency of the adjunct SMA staple fracture fixation constructs

Once the fracture is reduced, application of the SMA staple for interfragmentary compression is both efficient and reproducible. The procedure takes only a few minutes to prepare the staple insertion site and apply the implant. Efficiency of this technique is further improved during the application of the neutralization construct. Translation of the provisional fracture reduction into the definitive fixation construct can then be efficiently achieved with a neutralization plate. The plates' purpose is to protect the reduction and interfragmentary compression achieved with the SMA implant.

A locked plate can be applied to the bone as an internal fixator which is often less time consuming and less dependent on a perfect plate contour compared to a compression plate construct.

OUTCOMES OF SHAPE-MEMORY ALLOY STAPLES USED FOR FRACTURE FIXATION

Only two publications have reported nitinol staple fixation of fractures. In 1987, Yang and colleagues[15] reported 10 ankle fractures, 2 patellar fractures, 2 olecranon fractures, and 7 metacarpal and phalangeal fractures with isolated staple fixation without any neutralization construct. Other uses of SMA staples in their series included wrist, foot and hip arthrodesis, osteotomies of various bones and re-attachment of the peroneus longus tendon and medial collateral ligament. All fractures healed satisfactorily, with full range of motion of joints, except for 2 ankle fractures in which 5 to 10 degrees of

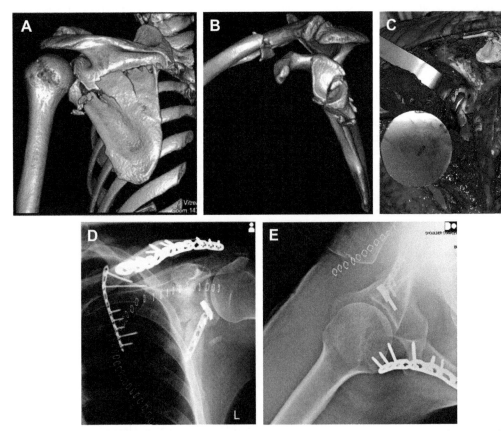

Fig. 1. (A–E) A 42-year-old man sustained a floating shoulder, distal third clavicle fracture and associated large inferior glenoid fracture extending transversely into the scapular body. An SMA staple was used for preliminary fixation to secure the large inferior glenoid fragment. Insertion of a lag screw perpendicular to the fracture would have been technically difficult due to soft tissue obstruction within the axilla. A neutralization plate was then applied along the lateral border of the scapula, and a plate was used medially to stabilize the remaining scapular body.

functional deficit remained. In patients who had follow-up of longer than 2 years, no signs of inflammation or tenderness were noted over the surgical site, and no radiographic evidence of staple loosening or bone absorption was seen. Eight patients had their staples removed (range 3–26 months after the initial procedure), and histologic evaluation found few inflammatory cells in the tissue surrounding the staples, supporting the idea that nitinol is highly biologically compatible.

In 1993, Dai and colleagues[16] reviewed 132 intra-articular fractures treated with only nitinol staples, without any additional neutralization fixation. Staples were used in 69 patellar, 43 malleolar (ankle), 15 olecranon, 4 lateral condylar and capitellar, and 1 tibial plateau fracture. All fractures were healed by 2 months. In 93 patients with follow-up of at least 1 year, none demonstrated clinical signs of late infection, local foreign body reaction, or radiographic evidence of staple pullout, breakage, or loosening. Nearly all (93.5%) of these patients reported excellent or good results. Seven patients had staple removal after fracture union, 4 because of articular protrusion, and 3 because of patient preference.

ADVANTAGES OF STAPLE FIXATION

There are many advantages of SMA staple fixation. These implants can be used to generate interfragmentary compression across fractures when traditional techniques are difficult or not possible. The posterior column acetabular and the glenoid fractures shown (**Figures 1** and **Figure 4**) have transverse fracture planes with respect to the surgical exposures. Orthogonal interfragmentary screw fixation across these fractures would require accessory percutaneous approaches that can be technically demanding. The SMA staples used for interfragmentary compression were applied through the same surgical approach and required only one c-arm fluoroscopy shot during insertion to prove the implants were in satisfactory position.

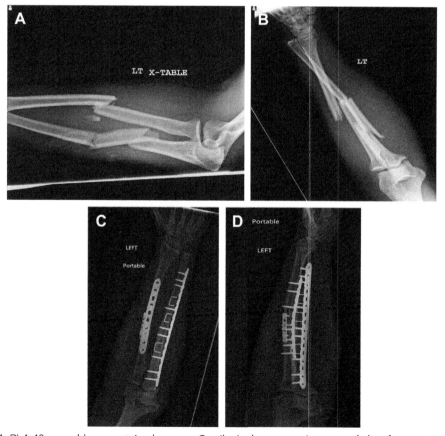

Fig. 2. (*A–D*) A 40-year-old man sustained an open Gustilo-Anderson type I segmental ulnar fracture, a transverse comminuted radial shaft fracture, and a distal radioulnar joint injury. After radial shaft fixation, the ulnar fracture fragments were sequentially held together with bone reduction forceps, and SMA staples were placed for provisional reduction and interfragmentary compression.

Staple fixation is also highly versatile, having small footprint instrumentation so these implants can be applied in spaces limited by soft tissues, bone reduction clamps, and other implants. This increases their appeal during the provisional reduction and fixation of fractures. These implants do not crowd bony corridors and can be applied quickly and reproducibly.

SMA staples obtains continuous interfragmentary compression and provides strong preliminary fixation with immediate continuous compression. This is in contrast to lag screw fixation, which is a static compressive construct that trends toward entropy.[18,19] SMA staple constructs may lead to greater stability, as these implants have the potential to maintain interfragmentary compression across the fracture throughout healing, despite fracture settling and bony resorption. As a result, SMA staple fixation may be biomechanically stronger than more traditional implants, especially when multiple staples are utilized[14,18,20] Furthermore, they can obtain uniform fracture compression even without purchase in the far cortex.[14]

LIMITATIONS OF STAPLE FIXATION

Despite the promise that these implants hold, there are several limitations to use of SMA staples. These include osteoporotic bone and highly comminuted fractures. Also, galvanic corrosion a concern when dissimilar metals are used in the same fixation construct. Lastly, these implants are currently associated with an increased cost when compared to traditional implants.

FUTURE DIRECTIONS AND CONCLUSIONS

Although the use of SMA staples as an adjunct in fracture fixation constructs is in its infancy, the implants hold promise due to the ease of application and simplicity of the technique, while facilitating and maintaining continuous interfragmentary compression. Cost-effective considerations, understanding where SMA staple compression can be optimized, and using proper indications are important factors for achieving consistent widespread success and minimizing failures. The use of nitinol staple implants will not likely not supplant traditional

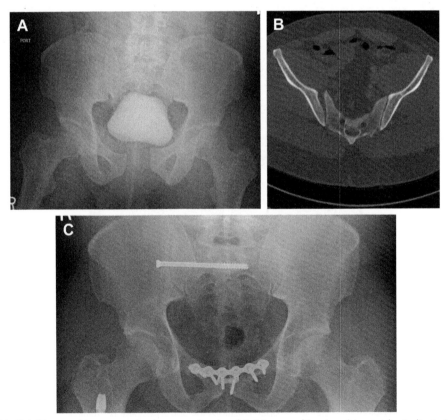

Fig. 3. (A–C) A 40-year-old man sustained an open-book pelvic injury resulting in pubic symphysis diastasis (type 2) and disruption of the right sacroiliac joint. An SMA staple was used as preliminary fixation to maintain compression and reduction while allowing reduction clamp removal, thereby permitting unobstructed plate application.

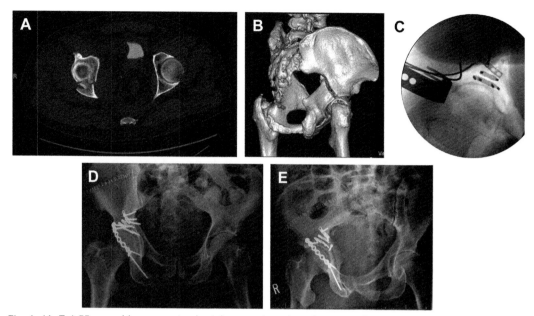

Fig. 4. (A–E) A 55-year-old man sustained a right posterior column fracture with an associated right hip dislocation. A posterior approach was used to expose the fracture, and SMA staples were used to compress and stabilize the fracture site with the aid of a buttress tubular plate to prevent shear during compression.

techniques for interfragmentary compression, however they may prove to be effective as another tool to the armamentarium in treating certain challenging fracture patterns.

CASE EXAMPLES

Case examples include

- Glenoid fracture (**Fig. 1**).
- Both-bone forearm fractures (**Fig. 2**).
- Pubic symphysis (**Fig. 3**).
- Posterior acetabular column (**Fig. 4**).

REFERENCES

1. Willmott H, Al-Wattar Z, Halewood C, et al. Evaluation of different shape-memory staple configurations against crossed screws for the first metatarsophalangeal joint arthrodesis: a biomechanical study. Foot Ankle Surg 2018;24:259–63.
2. Dunn J, Kusnezov N, Fares A, et al. The scaphoid staple: a systematic review. Hand (N Y) 2017;23:236–41.
3. Toby EB, McGoldrick E, Chalmers B, et al. Rotational stability for intercarpal fixation is enhanced by a 4-tine staple. J Hand Surg Am 2014;39:880–7.
4. Schnabel B, Scharf M, Schwieger K, et al. Biomechanical comparison of a new staple technique with tension band wiring for transverse patella fractures. Clin Biomech (Bristol, Avon) 2009;24:855–9.
5. Yaszay B, Doan JD, Parvaresh KC, et al. Risk of implant loosening after cyclic loading of fusionless growth modulation techniques: nitinol staples versus flexible tether. Spine (Phila Pa 1976) 2017; 42:443–9.
6. Driscoll M, Aubin CE, Moreau A, et al. Novel hemistaple for the fusionless correction of pediatric scoliosis: influence on intervertebral disks and growth plates in a porcine model. Clin Spine Surg 2016;29:457–64.
7. Buehler WJ, Wang FE. A summary of recent research on the nitinol alloys and their potential application in ocean engineering. Ocean Eng 1968;1:105.
8. Wang FE, Buehler WJ, Pickart SJ. Crystal structure and a unique Martensitic transition of TiNi. J Appl Phys 1965;36:3232–9.
9. Hodgson DE, Wu MH, Biermann RJ. Shape metal alloys. In: Davis JR, editor. Metals handbook. 2nd edition. Materials Park (OH): ASM International; 1990. p. 897–902.
10. Shenov A, Gordon S, Hayes W, et al. The Postsurgical stability of the nitinol shape memory staple in orthopaedics. FASEB J 2015;29.
11. Farr D, Karim A, Lutz M, et al. A biomechanical comparison of shape memory compression staples and mechanical compression staples: compression or distraction? Knee Surg Sports Traumatol Arthrosc 2010;18(2):212–7.
12. Bechtold JE, Meidt JD, Varecka TF, et al. The effect of staple size, orientation, and number on torsional fracture fixation stability. Clin Orthop Relat Res 1993;297:210–7.
13. Freeland AE, Zardiackas LD, Terral GT, et al. Mechanical properties of 3M staples in bone block models. Orthopedics 1992;15:727–31.

14. McKnight RR, Lee SK, Gaston RG. Biomechanical properties of nitinol staples: effects of troughing, effective leg length, and 2-staple constructs. J Hand Surg Am 2018;1.e1–e9. [Epub ahead of print].

15. Yang PJ, Zhang YF, Ge MZ, et al. Internal fixation with Ni-Ti shape memory allow compressive staples in orthopedic surgery. A review of 51 cases. Chin Med J (Engl) 1987;200:712–4.

16. Dai KR, Hou XK, Sun YH, et al. Treatment of intra-articular fractures with shape memory compression staples. Injury 1993;24:651–5.

17. Weber BG. AO Masters' Cases—Minimax Fracture Fixation. 1st edition. Dü bendorf, Switzerland: AO Publishing; 2004.

18. Hoon QJ, Pelletier MH, Christou C, et al. Biomechanical evaluation of shape-memory alloy staples for internal fixation—an in vitro study. J Exp Orthop 2016;3:19.

19. Kildow BJ, Gross CE, Adams SD, et al. Measurement of nitinol recovery distance using pseudoelastic intramedullary nails for tibiotalocalcaneal arthrodesis. Foot Ankle Spec 2016;9:494–9.

20. Lai A, Christou C, Bailey C, et al. Biomechanical comparison of pin and ninitol bone staple fixation to pin and tension band wire fixation for the stabilization of canine olecranon osteotomies. Vet Comp Orthop Traumatol 2017;30: 324–30.

Shoulder and Elbow

Lower Trapezius Tendon Transfer for Massive Irreparable Rotator Cuff Tears

Laura E. Stoll, MD[a],*, Jason L. Codding, MD[b]

KEYWORDS

- Irreparable rotator cuff tear • Massive posterosuperior rotator cuff tear
- Lower trapezius transfer • Arthroscopic tendon transfer • Shoulder external rotation

KEY POINTS

- Lower trapezius transfer has recently been described to restore function and provide pain relief in patients with massive, irreparable posterosuperior rotator cuff tears.
- An intact subscapularis or a reparable subscapularis tear is a prerequisite for a successful outcome.
- The lower trapezius is an in-phase transfer, which facilitates rehabilitation.
- The identification of the inferior edge of the lower trapezius muscle is key to harvest.

INTRODUCTION

There is no single definition of a massive rotator cuff tear. Descriptions includes those involving greater than or equal to 2 tendons, tears greater than 5 cm in width, or are based on the combination of tendons involved.[1–3] Although the term "irreparable" is somewhat subjective and a consensus for its definition has not been agreed on, irreparable tears often have significant retraction, poor tendon quality, fatty infiltration (Goutallier greater than or equal to III/IV), and muscular atrophy (Fig. 1).[4–8] These tears often cause significant pain and weakness. Although reverse shoulder arthroplasty is a viable treatment option in the elderly low-demand patient, treatment options for young and active patients are more limited. Attempts at repair, including partial repair, are challenging, and retear rates of 79% or greater have been reported.[9–13] Repair with bridging grafts has been described with some success, but it is an off-label indication according to the US Food and Drug Administration.[14–20] Superior capsular reconstruction is a newer technique with no long-term data available.[21–23] Debridement with biceps tenotomy can help with pain relief, but does not restore strength, and results tend to deteriorate over time.[24,25] Subacromial balloon arthroplasty is still in its infancy and its success is yet to be determined.[26] Latissimus dorsi tendon transfers have shown improved pain and outcome scores, but the transfer is out of phase, and outcomes are worse with subscapularis or deltoid insufficiency, as well as fatty infiltration of the teres minor.[27–30] This situation has led surgeons to investigate other muscle–tendon units for tendon transfer in patients with massive irreparable posterosuperior rotator cuff tears.

A lower trapezius tendon transfer was initially described as a successful treatment for restoration of external rotation in the paralytic shoulder.[31] It was later described as a treatment option for massive irreparable rotator cuff repairs.[32] The lower trapezius tendon originates along the spine around the level of T4, traveling inferiorly down to T12. It inserts 3 to 4 cm lateral to the medial spine of the scapula. It receives its

Disclosure Statement: The authors have no disclosures.
[a] Division of Orthopaedic Surgery and Sports Medicine, Virginia Mason Medical Center, 1100 Ninth Avenue, X6-ORT, Seattle, WA 98101, USA; [b] Department of Orthopaedic Surgery, The Everett Clinic, 3901 Hoyt Avenue, Everett, WA 98201, USA
* Corresponding author.
E-mail address: Laura.Stoll@virginiamason.org

Orthop Clin N Am 50 (2019) 375–382
https://doi.org/10.1016/j.ocl.2019.03.004
0030-5898/19/© 2019 Elsevier Inc. All rights reserved.

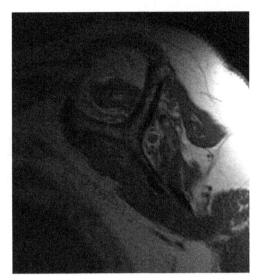

Fig. 1. Sagittal T1-weighted MRI image showing Goutallier grade IV fatty atrophy of the supraspinatus, infraspinatus, and teres minor muscles, representing an irreparable rotator cuff tear.

blood supply from the transverse cervical artery and innervation from the spinal accessory nerve (cranial nerve XI).[33]

Compared with the latissimus dorsi tendon transfer, the lower trapezius transfer has the advantage of being in phase with the infraspinatus, allowing for recruitment and ease of rehabilitation.[32,34] Additionally, the lower trapezius transfer has a similar line of pull to the infraspinatus, and excursion and tendon forces are more similar to the infraspinatus. Owing to the limited excursion of the lower trapezius tendon, it requires the use of an allograft or autograft to bridge the gap between the tendon and greater tuberosity. Both open and arthroscopically assisted techniques have been described.[35,36]

INDICATIONS/CONTRAINDICATIONS

Indications (**Table 1**)
- Irreparable massive posterosuperior rotator cuff tear
  - Goutallier grade greater than or equal to 3 for supraspinatus and greater than or equal to 2 for infraspinatus
  - Patte grade greater than or equal to 2
- Chief complaint of weakness, particularly external rotation

Contraindications
- Multiple medical comorbidities with contraindications for surgery
- Inability to comply with postoperative instructions

Table 1 Indications and contraindications to lower trapezius tendon transfer	
Indications	**Contraindications**
Massive irreparable posterosuperior rotator cuff tear Chief complaint of weakness, particularly external rotation with arm at side	Multiple medical comorbidities with contraindications to surgery Inability to comply with postoperative instructions Advanced glenohumeral arthritis Advanced age Subscapularis deficiency Deltoid deficiency Trapezius deficiency Forward elevation <60° (relative contraindication)

- Advanced glenohumeral joint arthritis
- Advanced age
- Subscapularis deficiency
- Deltoid deficiency
- Trapezius deficiency
- Forward elevation of less than 60° (relative contraindication)

SURGICAL TECHNIQUE/PROCEDURE
Preoperative Planning
A detailed history and physical examination must be obtained to determine the patient's goals and ascertain if they are a candidate for a tendon transfer. Plain radiographs and an MRI should be obtained with every patient.

Key factors in the patient's history

- Previous rotator cuff repair
- Chronicity of the injury
- Age
- Medical comorbidities including diabetes and immunosuppression
- Tobacco use
- Social and occupational demands
- Determining whether pain or lack of function/weakness is the biggest concern

Key factors in the patient's examination

- Forward elevation, abduction, and external rotation range of motion and strength
- External rotation lag signs and horn blower test
- Atrophy in the supraspinatus and infraspinatus fossae

- Subscapularis testing (belly press test, lift-off test)
- Deltoid testing
- Trapezius and serratus anterior strength testing and any signs of atrophy or dysfunction

Radiograph factors to assess

- Glenohumeral arthritis
- Humeral head elevation and acetabularization of the acromion

MRI factors to assess

- Rotator cuff tendon retraction, tendon length, and associated fatty atrophy of the muscle bellies
- Pay particular attention to the integrity of the subscapularis, because a functioning subscapularis may be needed for a successful functional outcome

Preparation and Patient Positioning

- The procedure is done under general anesthesia.
- The patient is positioned in either the beach-chair or lateral decubitus position, depending on the surgeon's preference.
- The patient must be draped such that the medial scapular border can be easily accessed.
- Arm holders can be useful to hold the arm in the appropriate position during tendon harvest and attachment.
- The spine of the scapula, medial border of the scapula, and origin of the trapezius are marked out.

Surgical Approach

- The original technique describes an acromial osteotomy. The arthroscopic-assisted technique was developed as an attempt to avoid the acromial osteotomy or violation of the deltoid for exposure of the greater tuberosity. The approach for tendon harvest is the same in both techniques.
- A vertical or hockey stick–shaped incision is made around the inferior scapular spine, starting 1 cm medial to the medial edge of the scapula extending to 3 to 4 cm lateral to the medial edge of the scapula (**Fig. 2**).
- Full-thickness skin flaps are created over the fascia of the lower trapezius and infraspinatus.

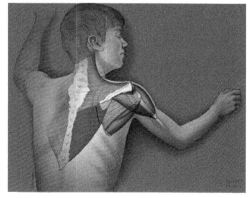

Fig. 2. The lower trapezius originates along the spine from T4 to T12. It inserts 3 to 4 cm lateral to the medial spine of the scapula. The harvest incision is made 1 cm medial to the medial border of the scapula. (*From* Clark NJ, Elhassan BT. The Role of Tendon Transfers for Irreparable Rotator Cuff Tears Musculoskeletal Medicine, 2018;11:141–9 used with permission of Mayo Foundation for Medical Education and Research, all rights reserved.)

- The lower trapezius muscle fibers travel toward the medial spine of scapula. The lower trapezius tendon forms a triangle. It is 23 mm in height and 40 mm in length.[36]
- The inferior edge of the muscle belly is exposed. The inferior edge of the muscle can be bluntly separated from the underlying infraspinatus fascia.
- Trace the inferior edge of the muscle to its musculotendinous junction and attachment of the spine of the scapula. A triangle of fat is usually seen in this area.
- The middle trapezius usually drapes over the lower trapezius and inserts more laterally onto the spine. A branch of the spinal accessory nerve to the middle trapezius can be encountered if the dissection is too superior.

Surgical Procedure
Tendon harvest

- Detach the lower trapezius tendon, including the underlying periosteum, from the spine of the scapula.
- Mobilize the lower trapezius muscle from the middle trapezius. A fat stripe defines this interval.
- Exert caution when dissecting the deep fascia, because the neurovascular pedicle lies 2 cm medial to the scapula on the undersurface of the muscle.
- If the medial spine of the scapula is prominent, resect the edge to prevent compression of the pedicle.

Prepare the tendon

- Weave No. 2 or No. 5 nonabsorbable sutures in a locking fashion (ie, Krackow stitch).

Prepare the allograft

- Place 2 No. 2 nonabsorbable sutures along the superior and inferior edges of the thick part of the tendon. Use of different colored sutures can aid in correctly positioning the sutures arthroscopically.
- Use a marker to mark one side of the graft as posterior.
- Place 1 tagging suture at the other end (thin part) of the tendon to help with tensioning.

Open transfer

- A Saber-type incision is made just medial to the lateral acromial border.
- At the origin of the middle deltoid, an osteotomy of the acromion measuring 5 mm in thickness containing the middle deltoid is performed with a powered saw. The lateral acromion is mobilized to expose the greater tuberosity and the rotator cuff. Alternatively, a deltoid split can be made off the posterolateral border of the acromion to avoid acromial osteotomy.
- The subscapularis is repaired if needed. Any healthy supraspinatus and/or infraspinatus tissue is partially repaired.
- The Achilles allograft is secured to the distal end of the harvested lower trapezius tendon either with nonabsorbable Krakow sutures or in a Pulvertaft weave (**Figs. 3** and **4**).
- A path is created deep to the deltoid through the infraspinatus fascia. The graft is then passed to the medial incision.
- Using bone tunnels or suture anchors, the graft is secured to the superior and anterior portion of the greater tuberosity while the shoulder is abducted to 90° and placed in maximal external rotation.

Arthroscopic-assisted transfer

- Perform a standard diagnostic shoulder arthroscopy. The subscapularis is repaired if needed.
- Establish portals.
  - The view from the posterior portal and work through the anterolateral and

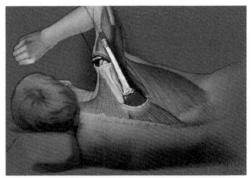

Fig. 3. An Achilles allograft is used to bridge the lower trapezius tendon to the greater tuberosity. A No. 2 or No. 5 nonabsorbable sutures are used to secure the allograft to the lower trapezius tendon. The Saber-type incision is seen with exposure of the greater tuberosity via an acromial osteotomy. (*From* Clark NJ, Elhassan BT. The Role of Tendon Transfers for Irreparable Rotator Cuff Tears Musculoskeletal Medicine, 2018;11:141–9 used with permission of Mayo Foundation for Medical Education and Research, all rights reserved.)

lateral portals to perform a subacromial debridement. Make the posterior portal more superior and lateral than usual to allow for better visualization of the tuberosity. Debride the footprint of unhealthy rotator cuff tissue until there is bleeding subchondral bone. Healthy rotator cuff tissue should be repaired or incorporated into the transfer.
  - View from the lateral portal. Identify the interval between the infraspinatus muscle belly and develop this interval using a combination of shaving and radiofrequency ablation. Stay intimate with the infraspinatus muscle belly to ensure that you are medial to the axillary nerve.
- From the medial incision, incise the infraspinatus fascia to create a path for the transfer (**Fig. 5**).
- Pass a grasping clamp from the anterolateral portal out the medial (harvest) incision.
- Pass the sutures attached to the Achilles tendon allograft out the anterolateral portal. This transfers the graft into the joint.
- Make sure the graft can easily move without any areas of restriction. Perform several cycles of shoulder rotation and graft sliding to ensure the graft moves easily. Visualize the marks on the posterior of the graft to ensure that the graft is not twisted.

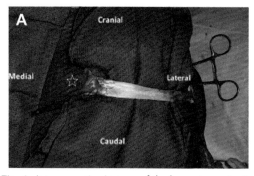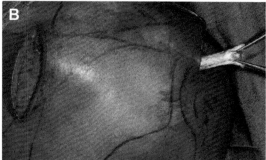

Fig. 4. Intraoperative images of the lower trapezius tendon prepared with the Achilles tendon allograft (*A*) before tunneling of the tendon and (*B*) after the tunnel has been passed deep to the deltoid.

- Anchor the graft to the anterior portion of the greater tuberosity using 2 suture anchors to incorporate the nonabsorbable sutures weaved into the tendon allograft.
- Place 2 preloaded suture anchors more posteriorly to further secure the graft.
- Place the arm in maximal external rotation and 90° of abduction.
- Split the medial aspect of the Achilles graft in half.
- Use a Pulvertaft weave to secure the inferior half of the allograft into the lower trapezius tendon. Oversew the superior portion of the allograft over the Pulvertaft weave.

Postoperative care

- A drain is placed if needed.
- Close each layer in a standard fashion.
- Apply an abduction–external rotation brace.

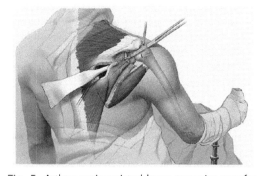

Fig. 5. Arthroscopic-assisted lower trapezius transfer. The allograft is first passed and anchored to the tuberosity arthroscopically. It is then weaved into the lower trapezius tendon with the appropriate tension. (*From* Aibinder WR, Elhassan B. Lower trapezius transfer with Achilles tendon augmentation: indication and clinical results. Springer: Obere Extremitat 2018, 13:269–272; used with permission of Mayo Foundation for Medical Education and Research, all rights reserved.)

Rehabilitation

- 0 to 6 weeks
  - Wear brace at all times. Elbow, wrist, finger range of motion.
- 6 to 12 weeks
  - Passive and active shoulder motion except no internal rotation.
- 12 to 16 weeks
  - Start gentle internal rotation.
- 16 weeks
  - Start gentle strengthening.
- 6 months
  - No restrictions.

Complications and Management

In Elhassan's original series of patients who underwent open lower trapezius transfers, complications included seroma formation, failure or stretch of the transfer, and infection.[32] The arthroscopically assisted approach is less invasive, and, therefore, theoretically has a lower risk of infection, less postoperative pain, and potentially faster recovery. In addition, it avoids the complications associated with a transacromial osteotomy, such as nonunion.

Outcomes

There are few published data on the outcomes of open and arthroscopically assisted lower trapezius tendon transfers given its novelty. In their original series of 33 patients treated with open lower trapezius transfers with a mean follow-up on 47 months, Elhassan and colleagues[32] reported improvements in pain, Disability of Arm Shoulder and Hand score, and the subjective shoulder value in 97% of patients. All patients except one had greater than or equal to grade 4 strength. Patients with greater than 60° of preoperative forward elevation had greater gains in flexion–abduction range. The external rotation lag sign, which was present initially in 82% of patients, resolved in all patients. There was mean improvement of 50° of forward elevation and 30° of external rotation. The 26 patients who showed preoperative proximal migration on radiographs had improvement in the mean acromiohumeral distance. Four patients developed a seroma. One patient required a glenohumeral arthrodesis after a persistent infection. One patient had failure of the transfer after a fall. Twenty-four percent of patients demonstrated incomplete healing of the acromial osteotomy, but this did not seem to affect outcomes.

Elhassen and colleagues[37] recently reported on 41 arthroscopically assisted lower trapezius transfers. At 13 months, 37 patients (90%) had improvements in all outcome measures. Pseudoparalysis resolved in 90% of patients. Final external rotation averaged 47°. Preoperative Hamada stage 2 and 3 changes tended toward worse outcomes. It is unclear as to exactly what preoperative factors predict a more favorable outcome. In a series of arthroscopic-assisted latissimus dorsi tendon transfers, those patients with lower preoperative outcome scores and a history of a failed rotator cuff repair had a greater likelihood of having a worse clinical results.[28]

Valenti and Werthel[38] recently reported on the use of semitendinosus tendon autograft instead of Achilles allograft in an attempt to avoid the potential complications associated with allograft. They performed arthroscopically assisted fixation to the humeral head using a cortical button and a bone tunnel. After a mean follow-up of 24 months, there was a gain of 24° of external rotation with the arm at the side and 40° of external rotation with the shoulder in 90° of abduction. Lag and horn blower signs resolved. Constant-Murley, the simple shoulder test, the subjective shoulder value, and pain scores all improved.

To date, there are no studies that suggest the superiority of latissimus dorsi transfer or lower trapezius transfer over the other. Biomechanical studies have suggested that the lower trapezius transfer is better at restoring joint reaction forces and glenohumeral kinematics compared with the latissimus dorsi transfer.[39] Hartzler and colleagues[40] suggested that the lower trapezius transfer is more beneficial for those patient who have limited external rotation with the arm at the side, whereas those patients who lack external rotation with the arm abducted to 90° would benefit more from a latissimus transfer.

SUMMARY

Massive irreparable posterosuperior rotator cuff tears present a challenging problem. The lower trapezius transfer has emerged as a reconstructive option in the young active patient to restore strength and function. Open and arthroscopic techniques exist. Long-term functional outcome studies are needed, but early results are promising.

REFERENCES

1. Gerber C, Fuchs B, Hodler J. The results of repair of massive tears of the rotator cuff. J Bone Joint Surg Am 2000;82(4):505–15.
2. DeOrio JK, Cofield RH. Results of a second attempt at surgical repair of a failed initial rotator-cuff repair. J Bone Joint Surg Am 1984;66(4):563–7.
3. Collin P, Matsumura N, Lädermann A, et al. Relationship between massive chronic rotator cuff tear pattern and loss of active shoulder range of motion. J Shoulder Elbow Surg 2014;23(8):1195–202.
4. Goutallier D, Postel JM, Bernageau J, et al. Fatty muscle degeneration in cuff ruptures. Pre- and postoperative evaluation by CT scan. Clin Orthop Relat Res 1994;(304):78–83.
5. Meyer DC, Wieser K, Farshad M, et al. Retraction of supraspinatus muscle and tendon as predictors of success of rotator cuff repair. Am J Sports Med 2012;40(10):2242–7.
6. Ohzono H, Gotoh M, Nakamura H, et al. Effect of preoperative fatty degeneration of the rotator cuff muscles on the clinical outcome of patients with intact tendons after arthroscopic rotator cuff repair of large/massive cuff tears. Am J Sports Med 2017;45(13):2975–81.
7. Kim JY, Park JS, Rhee YG. Can preoperative magnetic resonance imaging predict the reparability of massive rotator cuff tears? Am J Sports Med 2017;45(7):1654–63.
8. Gerber C, Schneeberger AG, Hoppeler H, et al. Correlation of atrophy and fatty infiltration on strength and integrity of rotator cuff repairs: a study in thirteen patients. J Shoulder Elbow Surg 2007;16(6):691–6.
9. Henry P, Wasserstein D, Park S, et al. Arthroscopic repair for chronic massive rotator cuff tears: a systematic review. Arthroscopy 2015;31(12):2472–80.
10. Heuberer PR, Kölblinger R, Buchleitner S, et al. Arthroscopic management of massive rotator cuff tears: an evaluation of debridement, complete, and partial repair with and without force couple restoration. Knee Surg Sports Traumatol Arthrosc 2016;24(12):3828–37.
11. Chen K-H, Chiang E-R, Wang H-Y, et al. Arthroscopic partial repair of irreparable rotator cuff

tears: factors related to greater degree of clinical improvement at 2 years of follow-up. Arthroscopy 2017;33(11):1949–55.

12. Kim S-J, Lee I-S, Kim S-H, et al. Arthroscopic partial repair of irreparable large to massive rotator cuff tears. Arthroscopy 2012;28(6):761–8.

13. Galatz LM, Ball CM, Teefey SA, et al. The outcome and repair integrity of completely arthroscopically repaired large and massive rotator cuff tears. J Bone Joint Surg Am 2004;86-A(2):219–24.

14. Pandey R, Tafazal S, Shyamsundar S, et al. Outcome of partial repair of massive rotator cuff tears with and without human tissue allograft bridging repair. Shoulder Elbow 2017;9(1):23–30.

15. Mori D, Funakoshi N, Yamashita F. Arthroscopic surgery of irreparable large or massive rotator cuff tears with low-grade fatty degeneration of the infraspinatus: patch autograft procedure versus partial repair procedure. Arthroscopy 2013;29(12): 1911–21.

16. Lewington MR, Ferguson DP, Smith TD, et al. Graft utilization in the bridging reconstruction of irreparable rotator cuff tears: a systematic review. Am J Sports Med 2017;45(13):3149–57.

17. Ferguson DP, Lewington MR, Smith TD, et al. Graft utilization in the augmentation of large-to-massive rotator cuff repairs: a systematic review. Am J Sports Med 2016;44(11):2984–92.

18. Lederman ES, Toth AP, Nicholson GP, et al. A prospective, multicenter study to evaluate clinical and radiographic outcomes in primary rotator cuff repair reinforced with a xenograft dermal matrix. J Shoulder Elbow Surg 2016;25(12):1961–70.

19. Steinhaus ME, Makhni EC, Cole BJ, et al. Outcomes after patch use in rotator cuff repair. Arthroscopy 2016;32(8):1676–90.

20. Ono Y, Dávalos Herrera DA, Woodmass JM, et al. Graft augmentation versus bridging for large to massive rotator cuff tears: a systematic review. Arthroscopy 2017;33(3):673–80.

21. Mihata T, McGarry MH, Kahn T, et al. Biomechanical effect of thickness and tension of fascia lata graft on glenohumeral stability for superior capsule reconstruction in irreparable supraspinatus tears. Arthroscopy 2016;32(3):418–26.

22. Burkhart SS, Denard PJ, Adams CR, et al. Arthroscopic superior capsular reconstruction for massive irreparable rotator cuff repair. Arthrosc Tech 2016; 5(6):e1407–18.

23. Mihata T, McGarry MH, Kahn T, et al. Biomechanical role of capsular continuity in superior capsule reconstruction for irreparable tears of the supraspinatus tendon. Am J Sports Med 2016;44(6): 1423–30.

24. Walch G, Edwards TB, Boulahia A, et al. Arthroscopic tenotomy of the long head of the biceps in the treatment of rotator cuff tears: clinical and radiographic results of 307 cases. J Shoulder Elbow Surg 2005;14(3):238–46.

25. Boileau P, Baqué F, Valerio L, et al. Isolated arthroscopic biceps tenotomy or tenodesis improves symptoms in patients with massive irreparable rotator cuff tears. J Bone Joint Surg Am 2007;89(4): 747–57.

26. Ricci M, Vecchini E, Bonfante E, et al. A clinical and radiological study of biodegradable subacromial spacer in the treatment of massive irreparable rotator cuff tears. Acta Biomed 2017;88(4S):75–80.

27. Gerber C, Rahm SA, Catanzaro S, et al. Latissimus dorsi tendon transfer for treatment of irreparable posterosuperior rotator cuff tears: long-term results at a minimum follow-up of ten years. J Bone Joint Surg Am 2013;95(21):1920–6.

28. Castricini R, De Benedetto M, Familiari F, et al. Functional status and failed rotator cuff repair predict outcomes after arthroscopic-assisted latissimus dorsi transfer for irreparable massive rotator cuff tears. J Shoulder Elbow Surg 2016;25(4):658–65.

29. Iannotti JP, Hennigan S, Herzog R, et al. Latissimus dorsi tendon transfer for irreparable posterosuperior rotator cuff tears. Factors affecting outcome. J Bone Joint Surg Am 2006;88(2):342–8.

30. Kanatlı U, Özer M, Ataoğlu MB, et al. Arthroscopic-assisted Latissimus Dorsi Tendon transfer for massive, irreparable rotator cuff tears: technique and short-term follow-up of patients with pseudoparalysis. Arthroscopy 2017;33(5):929–37.

31. Elhassan B, Bishop A, Shin A. Trapezius transfer to restore external rotation in a patient with a brachial plexus injury. A case report. J Bone Joint Surg Am 2009;91(4):939–44.

32. Elhassan BT, Wagner ER, Werthel J-D. Outcome of lower trapezius transfer to reconstruct massive irreparable posterior-superior rotator cuff tear. J Shoulder Elbow Surg 2016;25(8):1346–53.

33. Omid R, Cavallero MJ, Granholm D, et al. Surgical anatomy of the lower trapezius tendon transfer. J Shoulder Elbow Surg 2015;24(9):1353–8.

34. Smith J, Padgett DJ, Dahm DL, et al. Electromyographic activity in the immobilized shoulder girdle musculature during contralateral upper limb movements. J Shoulder Elbow Surg 2004;13(6):583–8.

35. Elhassan B. Lower trapezius transfer for shoulder external rotation in patients with paralytic shoulder. J Hand Surg Am 2014;39(3):556–62.

36. Elhassan BT, Alentorn-Geli E, Assenmacher AT, et al. Arthroscopic-assisted lower trapezius tendon transfer for massive irreparable posterior-superior rotator cuff tears: surgical technique. Arthrosc Tech 2016;5(5):e981–8.

37. Aibinder WR, Elhassan BT. Lower trapezius transfer with Achilles tendon augmentation: indication and clinical results. Obere Extrem 2018;13(4): 269–72.

38. Valenti P, Werthel J-D. Lower trapezius transfer with semitendinosus tendon augmentation: indication, technique, results. Obere Extrem 2018;13(4):261–8.

39. Omid R, Heckmann N, Wang L, et al. Biomechanical comparison between the trapezius transfer and latissimus transfer for irreparable posterosuperior rotator cuff tears. J Shoulder Elbow Surg 2015;24(10):1635–43.

40. Hartzler RU, Barlow JD, An K-N, et al. Biomechanical effectiveness of different types of tendon transfers to the shoulder for external rotation. J Shoulder Elbow Surg 2012;21(10):1370–6.

Ulnar Collateral Ligament Repair

A. Ryves Moore, MD[a,b], Glenn S. Fleisig, PhD[b], Jeffrey R. Dugas, MD[a,*]

KEYWORDS

- UCL • UCL repair • UCL reconstruction • Internal brace • UCL partial tear • UCL avulsion

KEY POINTS

- Ulnar collateral ligament (UCL) injuries are increasing in adolescent overhead athletes.
- There is a wide spectrum of UCL injuries ranging from partial tears and end avulsions to chronic attritional tears.
- UCL reconstruction has been the gold standard for treating all varieties of UCL injuries since Dr Frank Jobe performed the first UCL reconstruction in 1974 on Tommy John.
- Newer techniques of UCL reconstruction for partial tears or end avulsions have shown promising results with accelerated rehabilitation and earlier return to play compared with conventional UCL reconstruction.

INTRODUCTION

The anterior bundle of the ulnar collateral ligament (UCL) is the primary restraint to valgus force at the elbow and experiences tremendous stress during the arm-cocking and arm-acceleration phases of throwing.[1–4] With the increasing emphasis on sports specialization, year-round play, and ball velocity, UCL injuries have become increasingly common, most notably in baseball pitchers and other overhead athletes[5] (Fig. 1). Typically, rest from throwing activities coupled with rehabilitation is the first line of treatment.[6,7] If the athlete is unable to return to throwing after conservative measures, then surgery is recommended.[8–11]

Traditionally, UCL reconstruction as first described by Dr Frank Jobe in 1974 is considered the gold standard for the treatment of UCL injuries in overhead athletes.[8–10,12] Since UCL reconstruction was first described more than 40 years ago, the procedure has undergone technical improvements and has demonstrated better clinical results with regards to return to play and relatively low complications.[13–19] Despite this success, there are several shortcomings with UCL reconstruction. First, time to return to play is long (typically 12–18 months for baseball pitchers), meaning that athletes will routinely lose at least 1 season.[19,20] Second, given that these injuries are diagnosed in younger patients earlier in the injury process, it has been recognized that there is a wide spectrum of disease ranging from low-grade partial tears to chronic complete tears with tissue deficiency. This realization begs the question, is reconstruction necessary for the entire spectrum of UCL injuries, or is repair a viable option for some of these patients?

Historically, attempts at primary repair of the UCL demonstrated poor outcomes among professional pitchers, with 0% to 63% rates of return to play at the same level or higher.[8–11,21] However, recent reports of direct suture repair of an injured UCL have shown successful outcomes in young athletes with proximal or distal tears.[21,22]

Disclosures: J.R. Dugas is a paid consultant for Arthrex, Topical Gear, and Theralase; receives royalties from Topical Gear and Theralase; and has stock/stock options in Topical Gear and Theralase. No author or related institution has received any financial benefit or funding for this article.
^a Andrews Sports Medicine and Orthopaedic Center, 805 St. Vincent's Drive, Suite 100, Birmingham, AL 35205, USA; ^b American Sports Medicine Institute, 833 St. Vincent's Drive, Suite 205, Birmingham, AL, USA
* Corresponding author.
E-mail address: jeff.dugas@andrewssm.com

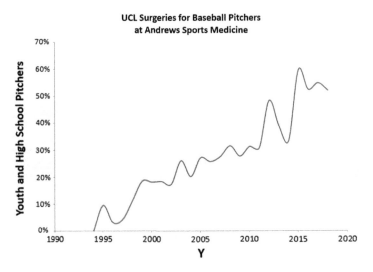

Fig. 1. Since 1994, UCL surgeries among adolescent pitchers have increased tremendously, especially in the last decade. (*Adapted from* American Sports Medicine Institute (ASMI). UCL Surgeries on Adolescent Baseball Pitchers. Available at: http://asmi.org/research.php?page=research&section=UCL. Accessed Feb 1 2019; with permission.)

Furthermore, at the authors' institution, they introduced a novel technique of UCL repair augmented with collagen-coated fiber tape (Internal Brace; Arthrex, Naples, FL, USA) to act as a backstop to valgus stress while the native ligament heals, allowing accelerated rehabilitation and faster return to play[23] (Figs. 2–4).

BIOMECHANICS

The anterior bundle of the UCL is the primary restraint to valgus stress at the elbow during the overhead throwing motion. Valgus loads during this motion have been analyzed and approach the ultimate tensile strength of the native UCL during the arm-cocking and arm-acceleration phases of the throwing cycle[1–4] (Fig. 5). There are several secondary dynamic and static stabilizers to the medial side of the elbow. If any of these are deficient, then increased stress is placed across the UCL, making it more susceptible to injury.

Despite abundant research on UCL surgical outcomes, there is a paucity of literature on the biomechanical data between UCL reconstruction and UCL repair. In a cadaveric study, Dugas and colleagues[24] compared the strength of UCL repair with internal brace augmentation

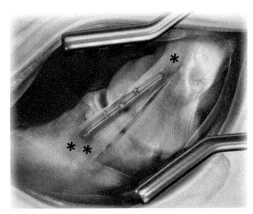

Fig. 2. UCL after repair with internal brace (Arthrex) was performed. Anatomic landmarks are labeled as proximal UCL insertion on the medial epicondyle (*asterisk*) and distal UCL insertion onto the sublime tubercle (*double asterisk*). (*From* Walters BL, Cain EL, Emblom BA, et al. Ulnar collateral ligament repair with internal brace augmentation: a novel UCL repair technique in the young adolescent athlete. Orthop J Sports Med 2016;4(3 suppl 3):2325967116S00071; and Arthrex, Naples, FL; with permission.)

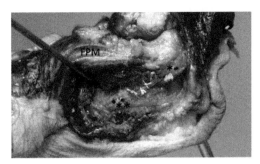

Fig. 3. Cadaveric specimen of UCL after repair with internal brace (Arthrex) was performed. Anatomic landmarks are labeled as proximal UCL insertion on the medial epicondyle (*asterisk*) and distal UCL insertion onto the sublime tubercle (*double asterisk*). FPM, flexor pronator mass. (*From* Walters BL, Cain EL, Emblom BA, et al. Ulnar collateral ligament repair with internal brace augmentation: a novel UCL repair technique in the young adolescent athlete. Orthop J Sports Med 2016;4(3 suppl 3):2325967116S00071; and Arthrex, Naples, FL; with permission.)

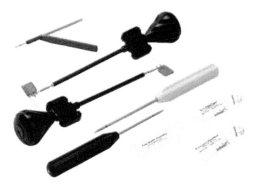

Fig. 4. UCL internal brace. Implant system (includes 3.5-mm PEEK [polyether ether ketone] SwiveLock, collagen-coated FiberTape, FiberWire, free tapered needle, 2.7-mm drill, drill guide, 3.8 mm tap and 3.45 mm punch/tap). (*Courtesy of* Arthrex, Naples, FL.)

to UCL reconstruction using the modified Jobe technique. They found that the augmented UCL repair replicated the time-zero failure strength of traditional graft reconstruction with respect to maximum torque to failure, torsional stiffness, and gap formation. When comparing UCL reconstruction to repair, they also noted that the repair was significantly more resistant to gapping at low cyclic loads (**Fig. 6**).

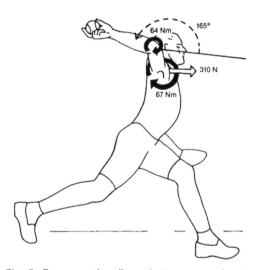

Fig. 5. Forces on the elbow during arm-acceleration phase of throwing cycle. Shortly after maximum external rotation is achieved, the arm is externally rotated 165° and the elbow was flexed 95°. Among the loads generated at this time were 67 N-m of internal rotation torque and 310 N of anterior force at the shoulder and 64 N-m of varus torque at the elbow. (*From* Fleisig GS, Kingsley DS, Loftice JW, et al. Kinetic comparison among the fastball, curveball, change-up, and slider in collegiate baseball pitchers. Am J Sports Med 2006; 34(3): 423–30; with permission.)

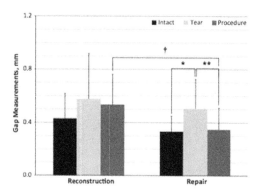

Fig. 6. The cyclic gap data for the repair and reconstruction groups. The repair group showed statistically less gap formation with small applied torque than did the reconstruction group ($^{†}P = .04$). Within the repair group, the torn condition experienced significantly increased gap formation compared with the intact condition ($*P = .04$) and a trend toward increased gap formation compared with the repaired condition ($**P = .07$). (*From* Dugas JR, Walters BL, Beason DP, et al. Biomechanical Comparison of Ulnar Collateral Ligament Repair With Internal Bracing Versus Modified Jobe Reconstruction. Am J Sports Med 2016; 44(3): 735–41; with permission.)

In another study, Jones and colleagues[25] compared the cyclic fatigue mechanics of an augmented UCL repair versus UCL reconstruction in cadaveric specimens. They found that after 10, 100, and 500 cycles of flexion-extension range of motion and applied valgus stress, the repair group exhibited significantly less gap formation as compared with the UCL reconstruction group. These studies show that an augmented UCL repair with an internal brace exhibits greater resistance to gap formation at time-zero when compared with the gold standard of UCL reconstruction.

INDICATIONS

Proper patient selection is critical for successful outcomes in UCL repairs. Typically, these are young, healthy, overhead athletes with proximal or distal avulsions or partial UCL tears that are unable to return to competition after a period of rest and rehabilitation. Also, there needs to be a vested interest in a shorter rehabilitation time in order for the athlete to return to play faster given specific time restraints and their specific goals. Most importantly, the UCL tissue needs to appear healthy on MRI as well as on intraoperative evaluation (**Figs. 7** and **8**). Those with poor quality tissue, such as that seen in chronic, attritional midsubstance tears, are poor candidates. Moreover, those patients with

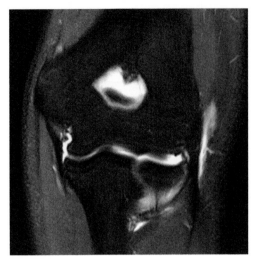

Fig. 7. Preoperative MRI with contrast of a pitcher with a distal end injury of the sublime tubercle. Note the intra-articular dye leaking out of the joint distally around the UCL insertion and into the surrounding flexor mass muscle belly.

large bony avulsions or ossicles within the UCL that when removed would compromise the remaining quality and quantity of the ligament are also poor candidates for repair.

TECHNIQUE

The first described UCL repairs were performed by direct suture repair with or without bone tunnels or with suture anchors.[9,11,21,22] However, the authors have developed a novel technique for UCL repair, which incorporates a heavy suture augmentation.[23] At the authors' institution,

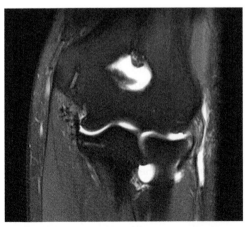

Fig. 8. Postoperative MRI with contrast of the same pitcher showing the healed distal end of the UCL injury to the sublime tubercle without extravasation of intra-articular dye.

UCL repair is done in a very similar approach to UCL reconstruction using a modified Jobe technique.

The patient is placed supine on the operating table with the affected arm draped out on a hand table. An examination under anesthesia is performed noting any preoperative range of motion restriction, particularly in extension.

- An approximately 6-cm incision is made beginning at the medial epicondyle extending distally.
- Ulnar nerve is identified and unroofed from the medial epicondyle proximally to the flexor carpi ulnaris (FCU) muscle belly distally.
- The nerve is mobilized without destabilizing it for visualization of the UCL.
- If the patient has ulnar nerve symptoms preoperatively, then the incision is extended proximally, and the ulnar nerve is fully dissected out from the arcade of Struthers proximally to the FCU muscle belly distally, and a subcutaneous transposition is performed using a 1 × 3-cm sliver of medial intermuscular septum as a fascial sling.
- The flexor muscle mass is then elevated off the UCL using a scalpel and soft tissue elevator.
- UCL is then split in line with its fibers from the sublime tubercle to the medial epicondyle.
- UCL injury is identified and inspected for tissue quality and for presence of any bony ossicles.
- Once the UCL injury is deemed appropriate for repair, the first 3.5-mm swivel lock (Arthrex, Naples, FL, USA) is drilled for at the site of the injury (proximal or distal insertion at the medial epicondyle or sublime tubercle).
- The hole is then tapped, and the anchor is inserted.
- The free suture attached to the anchor is then used to repair the ligament back to its origin in a mattress fashion with a free needle.
- The split in the native ligament is then repaired with 3 figure-of-8 stitches.
- The second drill hole is then made at the opposite end of the ligament and tapped.
- Tension is templated by aligning the third thread on the anchor with the aperture of the drill hole for the anchor. This would ensure that the joint would not be

overconstrained and extension would not be limited.

- The second anchor with the collagen-coated fiber tape is inserted and advanced to the aperture of the drill hole, while a varus force is applied and the ulnohumeral joint is held reduced in relative extension.
- The elbow is taken through a range of motion to ensure adequate isometry and tension of the internal brace. The ends of the suture are cut.
- The native ligament and internal brace are then sewn together with 3 simple stitches.
- The FCU fascia is closed with 1 to 2 simple stitches to prevent fascial incision propagation.
- The tourniquet is released, and hemostasis is achieved. If needed, a subcutaneous drain is placed to help prevent hematoma formation.
- Patient is placed in a soft dressing and a brace locked at 90° of flexion for 7 days to allow the wound to heal adequately for range of motion.

Patients undergo a UCL repair with internal brace augmentation physical therapy protocol, which is accelerated compared with the standard UCL reconstruction protocol. Patients typically begin plyometric exercises at 6 weeks once full elbow range of motion is achieved. A throwing program is initiated after 4 weeks of plyometrics. The athlete then can gradually return to full throwing by 16 to 18 weeks with the goal of being cleared to return to throwing in competition by 6 months.

Complications have included the following[23]:

- Ulnar nerve compression or instability: Despite requiring a secondary procedure, these patients' symptoms are easily alleviated with an ulnar nerve decompression and transposition.
- Heterotopic bone formation: In this instance, the patient required excision of the heterotopic bone on 2 occasions, with a season of pitching in between procedures. No routine heterotopic ossification is prescribed. However, a subcutaneous drain is placed to prevent hematoma formation in certain cases.

OUTCOMES

Initial data on UCL repairs demonstrated poor outcomes and dismal rates of return to play. Norwood and colleagues[11] first reported 4 patients who underwent UCL repairs in 1981, in which 2 of the 4 were able to return to sport. A decade later, Conway and colleagues[9] reported more than 70 UCL repairs and reconstructions. Of these, 14 underwent a direct repair of the ligament to bone in which 7 of them were able to return to their same level of play. In their subanalysis of Major League Baseball players, only 29% (2/7) were able to return to professional baseball, whereas 75% (12/16) of the professional baseball players who underwent UCL reconstruction were able to return to the same level of play.[9]

Because of these poor results and the positive outcomes and advances of UCL reconstruction, little investigation into UCL repairs was performed over the next 15 years. However, in 2006, Argo and colleagues[21] published promising results of UCL repairs in female athletes, in which 16/17 were able to return to softball, gymnastics, and tennis with an average return to play of approximately 3 months. Two years later, Savoie and colleagues[22] reported their results of direct repair on distal or proximal end UCL injuries on 60 overhead athletes. These athletes reported 93% good to excellent outcomes and 97% returned to play at the same level or higher.

Then, in 2016, the novel technique of UCL repair with internal brace augmentation was introduced by Dr Dugas and colleagues (**Fig. 9**).[26] Their initial retrospective study included 22 high-school-level athletes with proximal or distal injuries, except for 1 athlete who had a midsubstance ligament tear. All athletes progressed at the expected time interval with

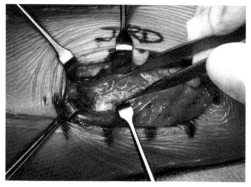

Fig. 9. Intraoperative photograph of UCL repair with internal brace (Arthrex) overlying repaired ligament. (*From* Dugas JR, Looze CA, Jones CM, et al. Ulnar collateral ligament repair with internal brace augmentation in amateur overhead throwing athletes. Orthop J Sports Med 2018;6(7 suppl4):2325967118S00084 and Courtesy of Arthrex, Inc., Naples, FL.)

Table 1
Subgroup analysis of functional score and time to return to play

	N	Analysis of Subgroups KJOC	P Value	RTP (wk)	P Value
Location of tear					
Distal	52	87.1	—	28.6	—
Proximal	55	88.2	.7	28.7	.9
Severity of tear					
Partial	63	88.8	—	28.1	—
Complete	43	86.3	.4	29.3	.5
Ulnar nerve transposition					
UNT	53	86.1	—	29.7	—
No UNT	55	89.1	.3	27.7	.3
Position					
Baseball pitcher	87	88.0	—	29.2	—
Baseball non-pitcher	12	81.2	.4	28.5	.8
KJOC score					
1 y	73	86.2	—	—	—
2 y	50	91.1	.04	—	—

Abbreviations: KJOC, Kerlan-Jobe Orthopaedic Clinic score; RTP, return to play; UNT, ulnar nerve transposition.

From Dugas JR, Looze CA, Capogna B, et al. Ulnar collateral ligament repair with collagen-dipped fibertape augmentation in overhead throwing athletes. Am J Sports Med; 2019; with permission.

rehabilitation and returned to competition at the same level or higher at an average of 21 weeks. All patients exhibited improved Kerlan-Jobe Orthopaedic Clinic (KJOC) scores, and 96% of the athletes were satisfied at 1 year.[26] More recently, Dugas and colleagues[27] presented a prospective study of 56 overhead athletes undergoing UCL repair with internal brace in which 96% of the athletes returned to sport at the same level or higher at an average of 6.1 months, whereas 65% were able to return to play in less than 6 months. All patients showed improvements in KJOC scores. In a follow-up study to their initial investigation, Dugas and colleagues demonstrated similar results in the first 111 patients who underwent UCL repair with internal brace augmentation at the authors' institution (Table 1).[23] These more recent studies demonstrate that UCL repair is a viable option for the younger overhead athletes with healthy ligament tissue.[27]

SUMMARY

UCL injuries encompass a wide spectrum of pathologic condition from partial tears, end avulsions, traumatic injuries, to chronic attritional ruptures. Initially, UCL repairs had shown poor outcomes. With increased understanding of UCL injuries and proper patient selection, UCL repair can be a viable option in young overhead athletes, allowing a safe and faster return to play than the traditional UCL reconstruction.

REFERENCES

1. Morrey BF, An KN. Articular and ligamentous contributions to the stability of the elbow joint. Am J Sports Med 1983;11(5):315–9.
2. Regan WD, Korinek SL, Morrey BF, et al. Biomechanical study of ligaments around the elbow joint. Clin Orthop Relat Res 1991;(271):170–9.
3. Fleisig GS, Andrews JR, Dillman CJ, et al. Kinetics of baseball pitching with implications about injury mechanisms. Am J Sports Med 1995;23(2):233–9.
4. Fleisig GS, Kingsley DS, Loftice JW, et al. Kinetic comparison among the fastball, curveball, change-up, and slider in collegiate baseball pitchers. Am J Sports Med 2006;34(3):423–30.
5. Olsen SJ 2nd, Fleisig GS, Dun S, et al. Risk factors for shoulder and elbow injuries in adolescent baseball pitchers. Am J Sports Med 2006;34(6):905–12.
6. Barnes DA, Tullos HS. An analysis of 100 symptomatic baseball players. Am J Sports Med 1978;6(2):62–7.
7. Kenter K, Behr CT, Warren RF, et al. Acute elbow injuries in the National Football League. J Shoulder Elbow Surg 2000;9(1):1–5.

8. Azar FM, Andrews JR, Wilk KE, et al. Operative treatment of ulnar collateral ligament injuries of the elbow in athletes. Am J Sports Med 2000; 28(1):16–23.

9. Conway JE, Jobe FW, Glousman RE, et al. Medial instability of the elbow in throwing athletes. Treatment by repair or reconstruction of the ulnar collateral ligament. J Bone Joint Surg Am 1992;74(1): 67–83.

10. Jobe FW, Stark H, Lombardo SJ. Reconstruction of the ulnar collateral ligament in athletes. J Bone Joint Surg Am 1986;68(8):1158–63.

11. Norwood LA, Shook JA, Andrews JR. Acute medial elbow ruptures. Am J Sports Med 1981;9(1):16–9.

12. Thompson WH, Jobe FW, Yocum LA, et al. Ulnar collateral ligament reconstruction in athletes: muscle-splitting approach without transposition of the ulnar nerve. J Shoulder Elbow Surg 2001;10(2): 152–7.

13. Dodson CC, Thomas A, Dines JS, et al. Medial ulnar collateral ligament reconstruction of the elbow in throwing athletes. Am J Sports Med 2006;34(12): 1926–32.

14. Paletta GA Jr, Wright RW. The modified docking procedure for elbow ulnar collateral ligament reconstruction: 2-year follow-up in elite throwers. Am J Sports Med 2006;34(10):1594–8.

15. Koh JL, Schafer MF, Keuter G, et al. Ulnar collateral ligament reconstruction in elite throwing athletes. Arthroscopy 2006;22(11):1187–91.

16. Dines JS, ElAttrache NS, Conway JE, et al. Clinical outcomes of the DANE TJ technique to treat ulnar collateral ligament insufficiency of the elbow. Am J Sports Med 2007;35(12):2039–44.

17. Bowers AL, Dines JS, Dines DM, et al. Elbow medial ulnar collateral ligament reconstruction: clinical relevance and the docking technique. J Shoulder Elbow Surg 2010;19(2 Suppl):110–7.

18. Hechtman KS, Zvijac JE, Wells ME, et al. Long-term results of ulnar collateral ligament reconstruction in throwing athletes based on a hybrid technique. Am J Sports Med 2011;39(2):342–7.

19. Cain EL Jr, Andrews JR, Dugas JR, et al. Outcome of ulnar collateral ligament reconstruction of the elbow in 1281 athletes: results in 743 athletes with minimum 2-year follow-up. Am J Sports Med 2010;38(12):2426–34.

20. Makhni EC, Lee RW, Morrow ZS, et al. Performance, return to competition, and reinjury after Tommy John Surgery in Major League Baseball pitchers: a review of 147 cases. Am J Sports Med 2014;42(6):1323–32.

21. Argo D, Trenhaile SW, Savoie FH 3rd, et al. Operative treatment of ulnar collateral ligament insufficiency of the elbow in female athletes. Am J Sports Med 2006;34(3):431–7.

22. Savoie FH 3rd, Trenhaile SW, Roberts J, et al. Primary repair of ulnar collateral ligament injuries of the elbow in young athletes: a case series of injuries to the proximal and distal ends of the ligament. Am J Sports Med 2008;36(6):1066–72.

23. Dugas JR, Looze CA, Capogna B, et al. Ulnar Collateral ligament repair with collagen-dipped fibertape augmentation in overhead throwing athletes. Am J Sports Med 2019. https://doi.org/10.1177/0363546519833684.

24. Dugas JR, Walters BL, Beason DP, et al. Biomechanical comparison of ulnar collateral ligament repair with internal bracing versus modified Jobe reconstruction. Am J Sports Med 2016;44(3):735–41.

25. Jones CM, Beason DP, Dugas JR. Ulnar collateral ligament reconstruction versus repair with internal bracing: comparison of cyclic fatigue mechanics. Orthop J Sports Med 2018;6(2). 2325967118755991.

26. Walters BL, Cain EL, Emblom BA, et al. Ulnar collateral ligament repair with internal brace augmentation: a novel repair technique in the young adolescent athlete. AOSSM Specialty Days Abstract 2016. AAOS Annual Meeting. Orlando, FL.

27. Dugas JR, Looze CA, Jones CM, et al. Ulnar collateral ligament repair in amatuer overhead throwing athletes. AOSSM Annual Meeting, 2018. San Diego, CA.

Foot and Ankle

Nitinol Compression Staples in Foot and Ankle Surgery

Oliver N. Schipper, MD[a],*, J. Kent Ellington, MD[b]

KEYWORDS

- Nitinol staple • Shape memory • Dynamic compression staple • Hindfoot fusion • Midfoot fusion

---

KEY POINTS

- Nitinol staples are dynamic continuous compression implants unlike static mechanical compression staples, locking plate/screw constructs, and crossing screws.
- Nitinol staples recover plantar gapping and contact surface area after cyclical loading.
- Nitinol staples are simple and fast to implant.
- For midfoot and hindfoot arthrodeses, nitinol staples have a high radiographic fusion rate.
- New-generation nitinol staples do not require refrigeration to reach noncompressed state or heating to reach compressed state.

INTRODUCTION

Nickel titanium is a metal alloy more commonly referred to as nitinol, which stands for *Nickel Titanium Naval Ordinance Laboratory* after where it was developed in 1959. William J. Buehler and Frederick Wang discovered nitinol while attempting to create an improved missile nose cone. During a laboratory management meeting, Buehler brought a strip of nitinol that he folded into an accordion to demonstrate to colleagues that he could manually return the material to its original shape. Fortuitously, the associate director of the laboratory took out his pipe lighter in proximity to the nitinol strip, which caused it to return to its original flat conformation rapidly, thereby demonstrating the shape memory characteristic of nitinol. Nitinol was subsequently developed as a metal alloy and used in dental archwires in 1976 followed by F-14 fighter aircraft hydraulic couplings in 1978. Although the material has been available since 1959, it did not gain broader commercial application until the 1980s because of challenges with the manufacturing of nitinol.

Nitinol is a near-equiatomic nickel-titanium alloy that is biologically safe.[1] Slight changes in the ratio of nickel to titanium result in significant changes in the transition temperature of the metal alloy. It undergoes martensitic transformation, a reversible solid-state phase transformation characteristic of all shape memory alloys, between martensite (monoclinic crystal structure) at lower temperatures and austenite (cubic crystal structure) at higher temperatures.[2,3] Nitinol is also superelastic, capable of recovering its original shape without plastically deforming until it reaches approximately 7% to 8% strain, which is almost 40 times the capacity of stainless steel.[2,4]

Early generation nitinol staples released in the 1990s and early 2000s were hindered by the need for refrigeration to maintain the noncompressed state and/or heating (ie, electrocautery) to reach the compressed state. First-generation nitinol staples also demonstrated poor fatigue

---

Disclosure Statement: O.N. Schipper: paid consultant: DePuy/Synthes, A Johnson & Johnson Company. J.K. Ellington: IP royalties: BME; paid consultant; paid presenter or speaker: DePuy/Synthes, A Johnson & Johnson Company.
[a] Anderson Orthopaedic Clinic, 2445 Army Navy Drive, Arlington, VA 22206, USA; [b] OrthoCarolina Foot & Ankle Institute, 2001 Vail Avenue, Suite 200B, Charlotte, NC 28207, USA
* Corresponding author.
E-mail address: oschipper@andersonclinic.com

strength and a poor ability to resist plantar gapping with load compared with crossing screw and plate constructs.[5] New-generation nitinol staples have gained popularity as a result of ease and speed of insertion, as well as superelastic properties at human body temperature, allowing implants to deform and return to their original shape (ie, with weightbearing) without the need for refrigeration and/or other heating.[6,7] Clinically, new-generation nitinol staples are capable of undergoing a thermal conformational change from a noncompressed state to a compressed state with body heat, making them ideal for use in midfoot and hindfoot fusions, as well as certain trauma applications. Over time, the viscoelastic properties of bone lead to stress relaxation, which reduces initial static implant compression.[8,9] Nitinol staples are capable of maintaining continuous compression after implantation (dynamic compression).[10] As a result, nitinol implants will dynamically reduce and compress bone fragments together after implantation as bone resorption or settling occur until the implant reaches its fully unloaded conformation.

NITINOL STAPLE BIOMECHANICAL DATA

The most common nitinol implant used in orthopedic foot and ankle surgery is the nitinol staple. The basic staple design includes 4 points of fixation: the proximal cortices where the curvature of the staple contacts the bone and the distal cortices at the tip of the staple. This allows more even load distribution across the site of compression. Screws only have 2 points of fixation: where the screw head contacts the bone and at the tip of the screw. The compression footprint of nitinol staples also extends approximately 2 mm beyond the tips of the staple.[11] Therefore, bicortical placement of the staple may not be necessary as long as the tips of the staple legs are within 2 mm of the far cortex.

The ability to dynamically compress materials makes nitinol staples unique from simple mechanical static compression staples. An in vitro comparison of nitinol and mechanical compression staples using a Lapidus arthrodesis model demonstrated that nitinol staples had superior, continuous compression and no far cortex distraction, unlike the mechanical staples.[12] With mechanical loading, nitinol staples maintain time zero (time of insertion) initial contact force and contact area and showed a 7% increase in compression in the first 10 minutes after implantation, unlike plate and screw constructs in which

compression decreased over time.[10] Another comparison between nitinol staples and a standard stainless steel mechanical compression staple found that mechanical staples had a 4 times higher resistance to bending and torsion, but had permanent deformation (plantar gapping) with bending.[7] In contrast, the nitinol had complete recovery of plantar gapping after mechanical loading.

Many options exist for fixation for joint arthrodesis. Nitinol staples also have significantly higher compression and contact areas, but lower stiffness with regard to lateral bending before and after mechanical loading when compared with a simple bridge plate construct.[10] With regard to nitinol staple constructs, 2 orthogonal staples have demonstrated significantly higher initial contact force, stiffness, and peak load to failure when compared with a single staple construct.[13,14] A separate in vitro comparison of single nitinol staple, double nitinol staples, crossed screws, and claw plate constructs for first tarsometatarsal arthrodesis showed that claw plates had the greatest plantar gapping with load, whereas the crossed screw construct had the lowest plantar gapping with load.[15] Plantar gapping was not recoverable in the crossed screw and claw plate constructs, unlike the nitinol staple constructs. The double staple construct had significantly less plantar gapping with load when compared with the single staple construct. Also, both nitinol staple constructs had significantly higher contact forces before and after mechanical loading when compared with the crossed screw and claw plate constructs. The double staple construct had the highest contact forces.

Although countersinking is not necessary for nitinol staples, surgeons may choose to reduce staple hardware prominence by creating a trough for the staple in bone. In a sawbones model, troughing for a nitinol staple had no effect on nitinol staple compressive force.[11]

Given the ability of nitinol staples to maintain compression with mechanical loading, the authors believe earlier weight bearing is possible with nitinol staples compared with other traditional implant constructs, but further clinical studies are necessary to confirm that it does not increase the risk of nonunion.

NITINOL STAPLE CLINICAL DATA

Nitinol staples are indicated for forefoot (first metatarsophalangeal joint), midfoot, and hindfoot arthrodeses, base of the fifth metatarsal fracture fixation, transverse distal fibula fractures, transverse osteotomy fixation, and noncomminuted fracture fixation. Contraindications for nitinol staples are nickel allergy and comminuted fracture fixation. A relative contraindication is osteoporosis or poor bone quality, especially with smaller bone bridges caused by the strength of compression and risk of iatrogenic fracture or cut out of the implant.

Limited data exist regarding clinical outcomes with nitinol staples. A prospective study of 27 patients (30 feet) who underwent first metatarsophalangeal joint arthrodesis using old-generation nitinol staples with a double staple construct demonstrated good to excellent results in 86.6% of patients There was 1 nonunion with full, immediate weightbearing postoperatively.[16] Another case series of 10 tarsal joint fusions using old-generation nitinol staples showed radiographic union in all patients, with an average time to fusion of 7.8 weeks.[17]

NEW-GENERATION STAPLES OFFER ADVANTAGES SUCH AS EASE OF INSERTION, GREATER COMPRESSION, AND HIGHER FATIGUE STRENGTH

Schipper and colleagues[18] performed the largest and first clinical study in orthopedic foot and ankle surgery using new-generation nitinol staples. The purpose of this study was to determine the radiographic union rate after midfoot and hindfoot arthrodeses using a new generation of nitinol staples and to compare outcomes between a nitinol staple construct and a nitinol staple and partially threaded crossing screw construct. All midfoot and hindfoot joints were included in the study with the exception of the subtalar and tibiotalar joints. The study included 96 patients undergoing midfoot and/or hindfoot arthrodeses and found that overall 92.7% (89 of 96) of patients achieved radiographic bony union. These results were similar to those published using locking plate and crossing screw constructs.[19–22] In the nitinol staple group, 93.8% (60 of 64) of patients and 95.1% (98 of 103) of joints had radiographic evidence of bony union at final follow-up. In the staple and screw group, 90.6% (29 of 32) of patients and 95.7% (44 of 46) of joints had radiographic evidence of bony union at final follow-up. The study also found no significant difference between use of staples alone versus use of a nitinol staple and crossing screw together.

There were no deep infections, and 6.25% of patients underwent hardware removal for irritation. The talonavicular and naviculocuneiform joints had the highest nonunion rate; therefore, the authors recommend a minimum of 2 to 3 staples for arthrodesis of these joints (**Table 1**).

ADDITIONAL APPLICATIONS OF NITINOL

Indications for use of nitinol implants in orthopedic foot and ankle surgery are rapidly increasing as the technology improves with more available implants. Expanded indications include: pseudo Jones and Jones fracture fixation (**Fig. 1**), ankle arthrodesis (**Fig. 2**), tibial osteotomies (**Fig. 3**), tibia fractures, Lisfranc injuries (**Fig. 4**), double and triple arthrodeses (**Fig. 5**), and Lapidus bunionectomy (**Fig. 6**). Use of nitinol staples is appealing for trauma indications, because only a small incision is required and the periosteum can be well preserved other than small holes for the staple legs.[23]

Dynanail (Medshape, Atlanta, Georgia) was the first tibiotalocalcaneal intramedullary nail available with an internal nitinol element. The Dynanail internal nitinol element is pre-stretched (up to 6 mm) prior to insertion of the nail. After insertion, the internal nitinol element is released and returns to its original unstretched conformation, compressing centrally across the nail. Therefore, the Dynanail is capable of adding an extra 6 mm of compression after insertion to adjust for settling at the joint being fused or bony resorption. In a retrospective case series of 20 patients who underwent tibiotalocalcaneal arthrodesis with the Dynanail, the internal nitinol element generated an average of 3.5 mm of additional postoperative compression in the first 2 to 3 weeks after surgery (**Fig. 7**).[24] All 20 patients went on to union, but 2 developed a deep infection requiring further surgery.

Outside of orthopedic surgery, nitinol has various other uses, including cardiac stents, guidewires, catheter tubes, kidney stone retrieval baskets, and orthodontic arch wires.

SURGICAL TECHNIQUE FOR JOINT ARTHRODESIS USING NITINOL STAPLES
Preoperative Planning

Prior to surgery, one should consider patient bone quality and any prior hardware in place. Additionally, one should consider staple leg length and staple bridge width depending on joint being fused.

Table 1
Clinical outcomes

	Total Radiographic Union			Staple Only Radiographic Union			Staple and Screw Radiographic Union			
	Joints [N = 149]	Total Radiographic Union [N = 142]	Rate	Joints [N = 103]	Staple Only Radiographic Union [N = 98]	Rate	Procedures [N = 46]	Staple and Screw Radiographic Union [N = 44]	Rate	P-value
1st TMT	18	17	94.40%	12	11	91.7%	6	6	100%	.67
2nd TMT	35	35	100%	26	26	100%	9	9	100%	N/A
3rd TMT	18	18	100%	12	12	100%	6	6	100%	N/A
Lisfranc	4	4	100%	3	3	100%	1	1	100%	N/A
Intercuneiform 2	5	5	100%	3	3	100%	2	2	100%	N/A
Intercuneiform 2	1	1	100%	0	0	N/A	1	1	100%	N/A
Naviculocuneiform	8	6	75.0%	6	4	66.6%	2	2	100%	.54
Talonavicular	41	37	90.2%	24	22	91.6%	17	15	88.2%	.82
Calcaneocuboid	19	19	100%	17	17	100%	2	2	100%	N/A
Overall	149	142	95.3%	103	98	95.1%	46	44	95.7%	—

From Schipper ON, Ford SE, Moody PW, et al. Radiographic results of nitinol compression staples for hindfoot and midfoot arthrodeses. Foot Ankle Int 2018;39(2):177; with permission.

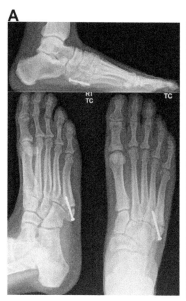
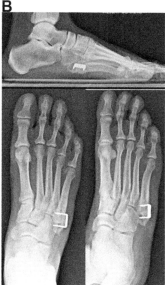

Fig. 1. (A) Preoperative imaging showing nonunion of base of the fifth metatarsal fracture. (B) Postoperative 6-week image showing healed base of the fifth metatarsal fracture.

Preparation and Patient Positioning

The patient is typically positioned supine with a bump under the hip and toes pointed toward the ceiling with the heel at the end of the bed in order to facilitate use of the mini-C-arm.

Surgical Procedure

For all joints, a longitudinal incision is made centered over the joint being fused using a #15 blade. Overlying neurovascular structures and tendons are identified and retracted. Dissection is carried down through the joint capsule. Meticulous joint preparation is performed using sharp osteotomes and curettes. Each joint is irrigated with normal saline. Both sides of the joint are fenestrated using a small drill bit. One to 2 cores of calcaneal bone autograft are harvested (optionally) through a small 1 cm incision over the lateral calcaneus posterior to the sural nerve and peroneal tendons using an 8 mm bone harvester. The joint is then reduced and held manually compressed or with a Kirschner wire. Optionally, a crossing 3.5 mm, 4.0 mm, or 4.5 mm screw may be used to hold joint position and obtain initial compression across the joint. For nitinol staple insertion, the drill guide (2-hole for 2-legged staples and 4-hole for 4-legged staples) is held in the desired position and checked under fluoroscopy. The 4-legged staple provides 8 points of fixation and therefore, higher strength, stiffness, and rotational stability when compared with the 2-legged staple.

All holes in the drill guide are consecutively drilled, and a temporary metal pin is placed in each hole. If the staple legs are too long, the legs may be cut to the desired length using a pin cutter.

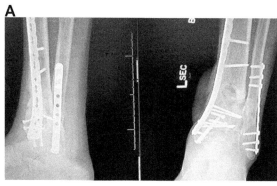
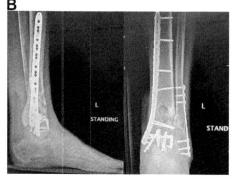

Fig. 2. (A) Preoperative imaging showing post-traumatic tibiotalar arthritis. (B) Postoperative radiographs showing ankle arthrodesis fixation using nitinol staples.

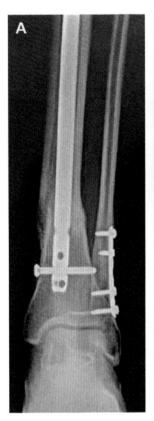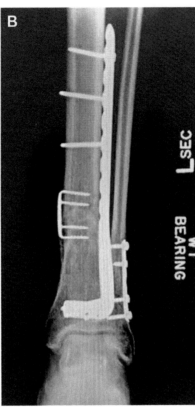

Fig. 3. Radiographs showing tibial valgus deformity (A) before and (B) after tibial osteotomy with hybrid plate and nitinol staple construct for fixation.

The guide is then removed along with the pins, and the staple is inserted into the holes. The staple is released from the insertion holder. Position is again checked relative to the joint prior to final seating of the staple down to bone. The staple is then tamped down until flush with the bone. Postoperative care based on the joint being fused is listed in **Table 2**.

COMPLICATIONS AND MANAGEMENT
Infection
Staples can be easily removed by first slightly elevating with a quarter inch curved osteotome and then cutting the central bridge with a heavy pin cutter.

Staple Breakage
Nitinol staples continuously compress bone fragments together, even as bone resorption occurs, and therefore may break late after surgery even in the presence bony union, although this is uncommon.[18] Nitinol staples are rarely symptomatic when broken.

Nonunion
In patients with persistent pain or evidence of staple breakage, a nonunion may be present.

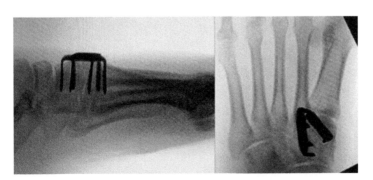

Fig. 4. Intraoperative fluoroscopy of unstable Lisfranc midfoot injury treated with nitinol staple fixation from the medial cuneiform to the base of the second metatarsal and second tarsometatarsal joint arthrodesis for instability.

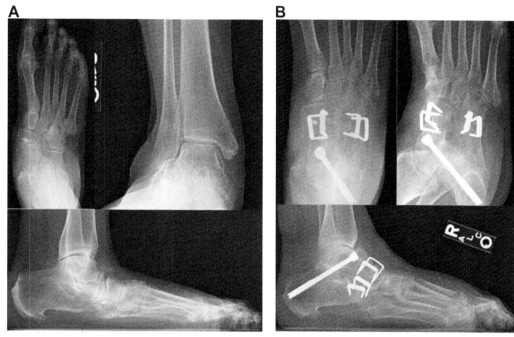

Fig. 5. (A) Preoperative radiographs showing severe planovalgus foot deformity. (B) Three-month postoperative radiographs showing correction of planovalgus foot deformity and fusion of the subtalar, talonavicular, and calcaneocuboid joints.

Computed tomography scan may be considered but can be challenging to interpret because of the small joint size and closely associated hardware. Radiographs are often easier to interpret.

Iatrogenic Fracture
Elderly patients with osteoporosis and patients with poor bone quality may be poor candidates for nitinol staples because of the strength of compression, which could cause iatrogenic fracture during implantation, especially with a smaller bone bridge.

Hardware Irritation
Most new nitinol implants are low profile, but they may cause irritation in areas with less soft tissue coverage.

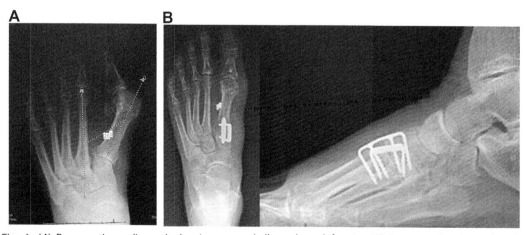

Fig. 6. (A) Preoperative radiograph showing severe hallux valgus deformity. (B) Postoperative 6-month radiographs showing correction of hallux valgus deformity via Lapidus bunionectomy with 90° to 90° nitinol staple construct.

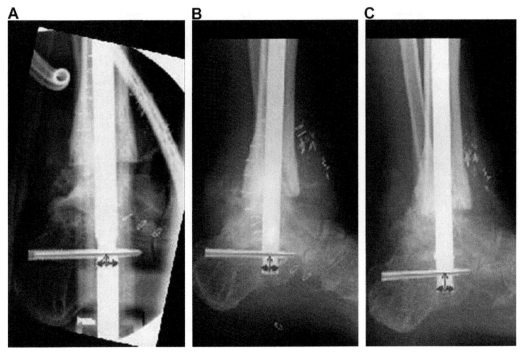

Fig. 7. (A) Intraoperative, (B) 2-week postoperative, and (C) 6-week postoperative lateral ankle radiographs showing dynamic compression secondary to the internal nitinol element of tibiotalocalcaneal arthrodesis nail.

		Table 2
Postoperative care		
Joint	**Staple Used**[a,b]	**Postoperative Weightbearing Rehabilitation Protocol**
First MTP	one 4-legged ELITE	2 weeks heel weightbearing
First TMT	one 4-legged ELITE	2 weeks non-weightbearing, 2 weeks heel weightbearing, then WBAT in cam boot
Second TMT	one 4-legged ELITE or one 2-legged ELITE	2 weeks non-weightbearing, 2 weeks heel weightbearing, then WBAT in cam boot
Third TMT	one 4-legged ELITE or one 2-legged ELITE	2 weeks non-weightbearing, 2 weeks heel weightbearing, then WBAT in cam boot
Lisfranc	one 4-legged ELITE or one 2-legged ELITE	4 weeks non-weightbearing, then WBAT in cam boot
Intercuneiform 1/2	one 2-legged ELITE	4 weeks non-weightbearing, then WBAT in cam boot
Naviculocuneiform	two 2-legged ELITE	4 weeks non-weightbearing, 2 weeks partial weightbearing, then WBAT in cam boot
Talonavicular	two 2-legged ELITE	4 weeks non-weightbearing, 2 weeks partial weightbearing, then WBAT in cam boot
Calcaneocuboid	two 2-legged ELITE	4 weeks non-weightbearing, 2 weeks partial weightbearing, then WBAT in cam boot

[a] In cases where there was inadequate space for a BME ELITE staple, a thinner bridge BME SPEEDTITAN staple was used instead.
[b] Surgeons may alter these constructs as dictated by patient bone quality and anatomy.

SUMMARY

Nitinol compression implants are fast and simple to insert, and have a high radiographic union rate for midfoot and hindfoot arthrodeses. Applications of nitinol technology in orthopedic surgery are rapidly expanding with the improved and broadened portfolio of implants available.

REFERENCES

1. Wever DJ, Veldhuizen AG, Sanders MM, et al. Cytotoxic, allergic and genotoxic activity of a nickel-titanium alloy. Biomaterials 1997;18(16): 1115–20.

2. Fernandes DJ, Peres RV, Mendes AM, et al. Understanding the shape-memory alloys used in orthodontics. ISRN Dent 2011;2011:132408.

3. Ramachandran B, Chang PC, Kuo YK, et al. Characteristics of martensitic and strain-glass transitions of the Fe-substituted TiNi shape memory alloys probed by transport and thermal measurements. Sci Rep 2017;7(1):16336.

4. Chang SH, Lin KH, Wu SK. Effects of cold-rolling/aging treatments on the shape memory properties of Ti49.3Ni50.7 shape memory alloy. Materials (Basel) 2017;10(7).

5. Neufeld SK, Parks BG, Naseef GS, et al. Arthrodesis of the first metatarsophalangeal joint: a biomechanical study comparing memory compression staples, cannulated screws, and a dorsal plate. Foot Ankle Int 2002;23(2):97–101.

6. Duerig TW, Tolomeo DE, Wholey M. An overview of superelastic stent design. Minim Invasive Ther Allied Technol 2000;9(3–4):235–46.

7. Rethnam U, Kuiper J, Makwana N. Biomechanical characteristics of three staples commonly used in foot surgery. J Foot Ankle Res 2009;2:5.

8. Manda K, Wallace RJ, Xie S, et al. Nonlinear viscoelastic characterization of bovine trabecular bone. Biomech Model Mechanobiol 2017;16(1):173–89.

9. Yakacki CM, Khalil HF, Dixon SA, et al. Compression forces of internal and external ankle fixation devices with simulated bone resorption. Foot Ankle Int 2010;31(1):76–85.

10. Hoon QJ, Pelletier MH, Christou C, et al. Biomechanical evaluation of shape-memory alloy staples for internal fixation-an in vitro study. J Exp Orthop 2016;3(1):19.

11. McKnight RR, Lee SK, Gaston RG. Biomechanical properties of nitinol staples: effects of troughing, effective leg length, and 2-staple constructs. J Hand Surg Am 2018. https://doi.org/10.1016/j.jhsa.2018.08.017.

12. Farr D, Karim A, Lutz M, et al. A biomechanical comparison of shape memory compression staples and mechanical compression staples: compression or distraction? Knee Surg Sports Traumatol Arthrosc 2010;18(2):212–7.

13. Bechtold JE, Meidt JD, Varecka TF, et al. The effect of staple size, orientation, and number on torsional fracture fixation stability. Clin Orthop Relat Res 1993;297:210–7.

14. Russell NA, Regazzola G, Aiyer A, et al. Evaluation of nitinol staples for the Lapidus arthrodesis in a reproducible biomechanical model. Front Surg 2015;2:65.

15. Aiyer A, Russell NA, Pelletier MH, et al. The impact of nitinol staples on the compressive forces, contact area, and mechanical properties in comparison to a claw plate and crossed screws for the first tarsometatarsal arthrodesis. Foot Ankle Spec 2016; 9(3):232–40.

16. Choudhary RK, Theruvil B, Taylor GR. First metatarsophalangeal joint arthrodesis: a new technique of internal fixation by using memory compression staples. J Foot Ankle Surg 2004;43(5):312–7.

17. Malal JJ, Hegde G, Ferdinand RD. Tarsal joint fusion using memory compression staples–a study of 10 cases. J Foot Ankle Surg 2006; 45(2):113–7.

18. Schipper ON, Ford SE, Moody PW, et al. Radiographic results of nitinol compression staples for hindfoot and midfoot arthrodeses. Foot Ankle Int 2018;39(2):172–9.

19. Cottom JM, Vora AM. Fixation of Lapidus arthrodesis with a plantar interfragmentary screw and medial locking plate: a report of 88 cases. J Foot Ankle Surg 2013;52(4):465–9.

20. Filippi J, Myerson MS, Scioli MW, et al. Midfoot arthrodesis following multi-joint stabilization with a novel hybrid plating system. Foot Ankle Int 2012;33(3):220–5.

21. Mann RA, Prieskorn D, Sobel M. Mid-tarsal and tarsometatarsal arthrodesis for primary degenerative osteoarthrosis or osteoarthrosis after trauma. J Bone Joint Surg Am 1996;78(9):1376–85.

22. Thompson IM, Bohay DR, Anderson JG. Fusion rate of first tarsometatarsal arthrodesis in the modified Lapidus procedure and flatfoot reconstruction. Foot Ankle Int 2005;26(9):698–703.

23. Singh D, Sinha S, Singh H, et al. Use of nitinol shape memory alloy staples (NiTi clips) after cervical discoidectomy: minimally invasive instrumentation and long-term results. Minim Invasive Neurosurg 2011;54(4):172–8.

24. Ford S, Ellington JK. Tibiotalocalcaneal Arthrodesis Utilizing a Titanium Intramedullary Nail With an Internal Pseudoelastic Nitinol Compression Element: A Retrospective Case Series of 33 Patients. Foot & Ankle Orthopaedics 2017;2(3). 2473011417S2473000171.

Anatomic Ligament Repairs of Syndesmotic Injuries

Craig C. Akoh, MD[a],*, Phinit Phisitkul, MD[b]

KEYWORDS

- Syndesmosis • AIFTL • PITFL • Tight rope • Deltoid ligament

KEY POINTS

- The resurgence of direct syndesmosis repair has attempted to address the shortcomings of syndesmosis screw fixation and isolated suture-button constructs.
- Biomechanically, ligament repair has been shown to be as strong as syndesmosis screw fixation.
- The quality of syndesmosis reduction seems to be the main factor for improving clinical outcomes after syndesmotic injuries.

INTRODUCTION

Isolated syndesmosis injuries are common in the competitive athletic population.[1,2] In the National Collegiate Athletic Association, the incidence is 1.00 per 10,000 athlete exposures, with 9.8% of injuries being recurrent.[1] The classic mechanism for isolated syndesmotic injures is external rotation of the ankle within the foot in a dorsiflexed and abducted position.[3] Syndesmotic injuries can also be seen in 13% to 20% of ankle fracture patterns,[4] including Maisonneuve fractures,[5,6] posterior malleolar fractures,[7] and bimalleolar ankle injuries.[8,9]

The ankle joint is a complex hinge joint that is composed of osseous and soft-tissue stabilizers. The primary osseous structures that constitute the ankle include the distal tibial plafond, talar dome, medial malleolus, and lateral malleolus.[10] The distal tibial plafond is concave in the sagittal plane and highly congruent with the convex talar dome. The medial and lateral malleoli are the distal most aspects of the tibia and fibula, respectively. Both malleoli serve as a buttress against medial and lateral translation of the talus. The incisura fibularis is a concave groove along the anterolateral distal tibia on which the lateral malleolus rests.[11] This groove provides the osseous stability of the syndesmosis.

Soft-tissue stabilizers are also important in maintaining syndesmosis stability. These soft-tissue stabilizers include the syndesmosis ligament complex and deltoid ligamentous complex.[12–14] The syndesmosis complex comprises 4 ligaments that maintain the distal tibia and fibula relationship, preventing diastasis. The anteroinferior tibiofibular ligament (AITFL) is smallest syndesmotic ligament, with a mean fibula insertion of 8.5 mm^2.[14] It is trapezoidal shaped, fanning out as it runs obliquely from the Chaput tubercle (tibia) and inserts onto the Wagstaff tubercle on the anterior distal fibula.[13] Posteriorly, the posteroinferior tibiofibular ligament (PITFL) originates at Volkmann's tubercle on the posterolateral distal tibia, running obliquely to insert onto the posterior aspect of the lateral malleolus. Its fibula footprint is 108.1 mm^2.[14] The inferior transverse tibiofibular ligament, also known as the deep PITFL, is a strong fibrocartilaginous structure just distal to

Disclosure Statement: The authors report the following potential conflicts of interest or sources of funding: P. Phisitkul is a paid consultant for Arthrex and Restor 3D, receives royalties from Arthrex, and has stock/stock options in First Ray and Mortise Medical. Full ICMJE author disclosure forms are available for this article online, as supplementary material.

[a] Department of Orthopedics and Rehabilitation, University of Wisconsin School of Medicine and Public Health Madison, 600 Highland Avenue, Room 6220, Madison, WI 53705-2281, USA; [b] Tri-State Specialists, LLP, 2730 Pierce Street, Suite 300, Sioux City, IA 51104, USA
* Corresponding author.
E-mail address: ccakoh@gmail.com

Orthop Clin N Am 50 (2019) 401–414
https://doi.org/10.1016/j.ocl.2019.02.004

the PITFL that runs in an oblique manner infero-laterally, similarly to the PITFL. The interosseus tibiofibular ligament is the broadest and most proximal structure of the syndesmosis, with a fibula footprint of 408.4 mm^2.[14] It represents the distal thickening of the interosseus membrane, terminating 9.3 mm proximal to the central plafond.[14]

The deltoid ligament complex, also an important soft-tissue stabilizing structure of the syndesmosis, is a fan-shaped structure that originates from the medial malleolus and inserts onto the navicular, talus, and calcaneus. Although the deltoid ligament is highly variable with up to 6 separate bands, it is constantly composed of the tibiocalaneal, superficial posterior tibiotalar, and deep anterior tibiotalar ligaments.[15] The deltoid ligament can also be divided into the superficial band, which originates at the anterior colliculus of the medial malleolus, and the stronger deep fibers that originate from the intercollicular groove and posterior colliculus of the medial malleolus.

Biomechanically, the syndesmosis ligamentous complex serves an important role in resisting tibiofibular diastasis and external rotation of the fibula, given the lack of osseous constraint of the syndesmosis.[16–19] Previous biomechanical studies demonstrated that syndesmosis diastasis was prevented with an intact deltoid during axial loading.[20] However, more recent studies have shown increased coronal diastasis up to 7.3 mm with sequential syndesmosis sectioning.[18] External rotation instability of the tibiofibular articulation is also increased when the AITFL and PITFL is sectioned by 24% and 11%, respectively.[16] The deltoid ligamentous complex is the strongest ligamentous structure of the ankle.[21] Both the superficial and deep fibers of the deltoid ligament complex must be intact to prevent valgus tilt of the talus and widening of the ankle mortise.[22] Sectioning of the superficial fibers of the deltoid ligament increases the peak contact pressures of the ankle joint by 30% and lateral translation of the talus by 4 mm.[23]

The classification of syndesmotic injuries has evolved over the years to predict outcomes and guide management. In 1984, Edwards and DeLee[3] described syndesmotic injuries as having frank diastasis, latent diastasis with stress examination, and no diastasis. In Amendola and colleagues' classification,[24] grade I was mild syndesmosis sprains, and grade II was moderate injuries with partial syndesmosis rupture, normal radiographs, and positive external rotation test. Grade II injuries can also be subdivided

into stable or unstable. Grade III injuries involve complete disruption of the syndesmosis with radiographic syndesmosis and medial clear space widening. However, the more subtle rotational syndesmotic injuries are often missed on plain radiographs.[25] With the improvement of advanced imaging, Sikka and colleagues[26] proposed an MRI classification incorporating deltoid injuries. Grade I injuries were isolated AITFL injuries. Grade II included AITFL and interosseus ligament (IOL) injuries. Grade III injuries involved the AITFL, IOL, and PITFL injuries. Lastly, grade IV injuries involved the AITFL, IOL, PITFL, and deltoid ligaments. MRI has been shown to be overly sensitive in detecting syndesmotic injuries.[25] Given the limited sensitivity of plain radiographs and overly sensitive MRI, intraoperative arthroscopy is becoming the gold standard for detecting subtle syndesmotic injuries.[25,27,28]

There are challenges in the treatment of syndesmotic injury using screw fixation, including malreduction, overcompression, screw removal, and hardware breakage.[29–33] The benefits of suture-button constructs are restoring physiologic syndesmosis motion,[34] reduced malreduction,[35] accelerated rehabilitation,[36] and less hardware prominence.[35,37] Despite these benefits, isolated suture-button constructs do not completely restore normal syndesmosis biomechanics.[38,39] In addition, complications such as skin irritation, implant loosening, and implant prominence have been reported.[40–42] Although there is limited understanding of direct anatomic ligament repair of ankle syndesmosis, advancements have been made in the surgical technique for syndesmosis repair.[43]

INDICATIONS AND CONTRAINDICATIONS

The indications for surgical treatment of isolated syndesmotic injuries continue to evolve with improved classification and understanding of these injuries. As a result, the fixation of isolated syndesmotic and syndesmotic injuries associated with ankle fractures has increased significantly.[8] The goals of syndesmosis surgery are to restore the normal anatomic relationship of the distal tibiofibular joint and to prevent ankle arthritis. Indications for surgical intervention for isolated syndesmotic injuries include frank syndesmosis diastasis or medial clear space widening on plain radiographs. Other indications include latent diastasis on stress radiographs or fibula malposition within the incisura fibularis during weight-bearing computed tomography (CT) imaging. However, there is no clear evidence for fixation of isolated grade II injuries without radiographic diastasis. There are suggestions that grade II injuries with significant disruption of the PITFL and deltoid ligament may be an indication for syndesmotic fixation.[24] Guyton and colleagues[44] showed that syndesmosis diastasis of 3 mm during arthroscopy correlated with significant syndesmosis injury. Patients who may benefit from deltoid ligament repair are those with medial diastasis or distraction after syndesmotic repair or those with complete rupture of both superficial and deep parts.

Contraindications to syndesmotic fixation include grade I ankle sprains without frank syndesmosis diastasis or grade II injuries without syndesmosis diastasis on stress examination without a trial of conservative treatment, except in athletes. Previous studies have shown that grade I and II injuries without diastasis can be successfully treated conservatively.[26,45]

SURGICAL TECHNIQUE/PROCEDURE
Preoperative Planning
There are several considerations that must be considered when planning the surgical management of syndesmotic injuries. Physical examination findings of positive squeeze test, dorsiflexion-external rotation, and inability to perform a single leg hop may indicate a more severe syndesmotic injury.[46,47] However, the absence of medial deltoid pain is not specific for the absence of deltoid injury.[48] The presence of blood-filled blisters may represent a deeper soft-tissue injury, and surgery should be delayed for 5 to 10 days.[49,50] Patient factors such as comorbidities, body mass index, and diabetes mellitus should also be considered. Less invasive fixation techniques can reduce would complication rates in the comorbid and elderly patient.[51,52]

Plain radiographs can assist in detecting frank diastasis of the syndesmosis and associated fractures of the fibula, medial malleolus, and posterior malleolus. However, plain radiography fails to detect subtle syndesmotic injuries[18,25,53,54] or bony avulsion injuries.[55] Boden and colleagues[56] previously stated in their cadaveric study that the level of the fibula fracture (greater than 4.5 cm from the ankle mortise) correlated with the presence of syndesmotic injury. However, the clinical study by Nielson and colleagues[57] showed that the level of the fibula fracture could not reliably predict the presence of injury to the syndesmosis. Thus, stress examination[48] and arthroscopic examination[25] should be used to determine the presence or absence of a syndesmotic injury. Standing bilateral CT

scans can be used to detect subtle syndesmotic malrotation.[53,58–60] A CT scan can also characterize the size and amount of articular involvement of avulsion injuries, which can dictate the surgical approach.[61] MRI can detect the extent of soft-tissue injury to the syndesmosis and deltoid ligament when frank diastasis is not present.[26]

There are several options for syndesmosis repair augmentation including metal screw and washer,[55] soft-tissue augmentation,[55] and suture-button contructs.[62] Syndesmotic screw supplementation may be considered for obese patients with marked syndesmosis diastasis. Length unstable fibula fractures should undergo fibular plate fixation in addition to syndesmotic fixation. Maisonneuve fracture should be reduced and fixed with rigid screw fixation to maintain anatomic rotation and length. Avulsion injuries of the AITFL (ie, Chaput or Wagstaff fragments) can be fixed with a screw-and-washer construct. The technique described herein focuses on direct syndesmosis repair and augmentation.

Syndesmosis Repair and Augmentation for Isolated Syndesmosis Injuries

1. The patient is placed in the supine position at the end of the operative table and the appropriate anesthetic method is administered.
2. Contralateral anteroposterior (AP), mortise, and lateral fluoroscopic views of the contralateral ankle are obtained for comparison of the operative syndesmosis reduction.
3. The patient is properly prepped and standard anteromedial and anterolateral arthroscopy portals are established.
4. Diagnostic arthroscopy is performed in the standard fashion to evaluate injury to the syndesmosis, deltoid ligament, and articular cartilage. Noninvasive distraction is typically not used unless osteochondral lesions are being treated.
5. If used, noninvasive distraction is taken off before syndesmotic evaluation. Using a 90° angled arthroscopic probe, the amount of diastasis seen in the distal tibiofibular joint is measured when the ankle is externally rotated to determine the amount of syndesmosis instability. A cut point of 3 mm can be used to indicate a definite injury to the AITFL (**Fig. 1**).
6. A 4-cm anterolateral skin incision is made centered on the distal syndesmosis. Care is

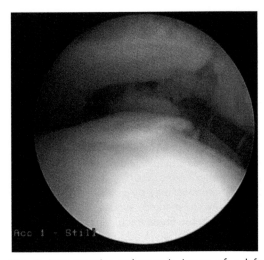

Fig. 1. Intraoperative arthroscopic image of a left ankle with significant widening of the ankle syndesmosis with probe palpation.

taken to protect the superficial peroneal nerve as it crosses the surgical field.

   a. Direct visualization of the syndesmosis leads to improved reduction.[63]

7. Ligamentous debris and scar tissue are removed to clearly visualize the injured AITFL.

   a. The location of AITFL injury should be determined (ie, bony avulsions versus midsubstance tear). Typically when there is no avulsion fracture, the AITFL is peeled off from the distal tibia to expose the ankle syndesmosis.

   b. Care should be taken to avoid injury to the perforating branch of the peroneal artery, as it pierces the interosseus membrane about 3 cm proximal to the tibial plafond.[64,65]

8. The injured syndesmosis is reduced under direct visualization usually by manually pushing the distal fibula in the fibular notch of the distal tibia along the neutral axis. Although the previous thought was to reduce the syndesmosis in dorsiflexion to avoid overtightening, this has not been confirmed in the literature, and the overcompression is less of an issue with flexible reconstruction.[66–68]

9. The reduction of the syndesmosis is provisionally held with pointed reduction clamps proximal to the tibiotalar joint if needed. The lateral clamp should be placed along the posterolateral aspect of the lateral malleolus. The medial clamp should be placed in the anterior third of the medial tibia. Careful placement of the

reduction clamps is important in avoiding malreduction of the syndesmosis.[69,70]

10. Adequate reduction is confirmed both directly and fluoroscopically. Direct evaluation involves ensuring that the distal fibula lies within the incisura fibularis and not anterior to it.[12] Fluoroscopy reduction confirmation is best seen on the lateral radiograph, with the fibula overlapping the posterior one-third of the tibia. The tibiotalar overlap and medial tibiotalar clear space is assessed on the AP and mortise views. If the tibiofibular overlap is inadequate, the reduction clamp is tightened further.

11. AITFL Avulsion repair

   a. If the AITFL involves an avulsion injury from the tibia (Chaput fragment) or fibula (Wagstaff fragment), the avulsed ligament is repaired directly at its origin by drilling and placing a screw-washer construct (**Fig. 2**).

12. AITFL Midsubstance repair

   a. If the AITFL injury is midsubstance there is often too much tension to allow for direct repair, and augmentation is used.

   b. The AITFL can be reconstructed using the fourth extensor digitorum longus tendon,[55] suture anchor-to-post construct[71] (described in the deltoid repair section) (**Fig. 3**) or suture tape construct.[72]

13. IOL Repair Supplementation

   a. Suture-button construct

      i. This step is a reconstruction of the interosseous ligament that is indicated for athletes and other patients with more severe instability in the central plane of the syndesmosis (**Fig. 4**).

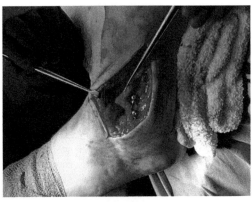

Fig. 2. Intraoperative image of a Chaput fragment avulsion undergoing anatomic repair.

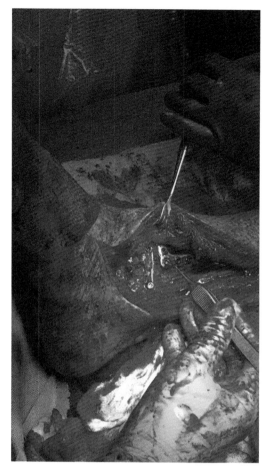

Fig. 3. The AITFL, which was previously peeled off, is repaired back to the distal tibia using a suture post construct.

ii. A drill hole is made at the posterolateral distal fibula 2 to 3 cm proximal to the tibiotalar joint. The drill hole should be made parallel to the tibiotalar joint at a 30° angle

anterior to the coronal plane to avoid intra-articular placement of the construct.

iii. The suture-button construct is then placed through the drill hole to provide trans-syndesmotic fixation. One should be sure to confirm the reduction directly and fluoroscopically once the implant is placed.

14. Deltoid repair

a. Ankle stability is reassessed with a gentle external rotation stress test. If medial clear space widening is present, a medial approach over the medial malleolus should be performed to remove incarcerated deltoid ligament from within the ankle joint and to perform a direct repair. Occasionally the medial joint space may appear widened after syndesmotic stabilization, indicating significant medial instability.

b. Pronation external rotation ankle injuries should be carefully scrutinized for medial clear space widening after appropriate fibula and syndesmotic fixation. Usually the superficial deltoid ligament is avulsed from its medial malleolus insertion.[73]

c. For acute deltoid ligament injuries, direct repair with suture anchor augmentation can be performed (**Fig. 5**).

d. For chronic deltoid ligament injuries with poor tissue quality, the deep deltoid can also be reconstructed using a suture anchor-to-post construct.[71] (see **Fig. 5**)

    i. A longitudinal incision is made over the medial malleolus and medial talus.

    ii. Soft-tissue dissection is made to expose the intercollicular groove of the medial malleolus and medial talus, taking care to protect the saphenous neurovascular structures.

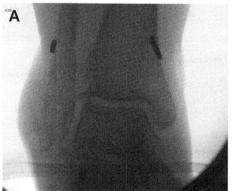
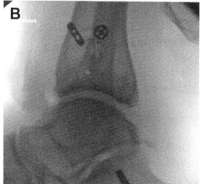

Fig. 4. (*A*) AP and (*B*) lateral intraoperative fluoroscopic views of a case of chronic ankle syndesmotic instability after previous syndesmosis screw fixation and removal treated with a suture-button construct.

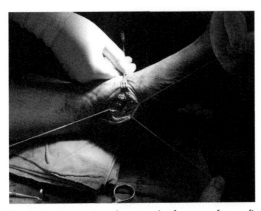

Fig. 5. Intraoperative photograph of a case of superficial and deep deltoid repair for a chronic medial ankle instability.

iii. The posterior tibialis tendon sheath is incised and retracted posteriorly to evaluate the deep deltoid ligament fibers.

iv. A small medial capsulotomy is made to evaluate for any interposed deep deltoid ligament fibers, and medial gutter debridement is performed.

v. A double-loaded nonabsorbable suture anchor is placed at the talar insertion of the deep deltoid ligament. Anchor placement is confirmed with fluoroscopy.

vi. A separate stab incision is made at the medial malleolus proximal to the tibial insertion of the deltoid ligament and a 3.5-mm screw-post and washer is placed in the medial malleolus.

vii. The suture limbs are passed through the deep and superficial deltoid fibers in a fan-like fashion and tied after fluoroscopic ankle reduction is confirmed.

viii. The suture limbs are then tied proximally over the screw-and-post construct.

ix. The posterior tibialis tendon sheath is repaired using absorbable sutures.

15. The wound is irrigated and the dermal and skin layers closed with interrupted sutures.

16. Dressings and short leg splint are placed over the operative foot to allow for postoperative swelling.

Syndesmosis Repair and Augmentation with Associated Ankle Fractures

1. The patient is placed in the supine position at the end of the operative table and the appropriate anesthetic method is administered. In patients with large posterior malleolus fractures, lateral or prone positioning may be considered to optimize direct fixation of the posterior malleolus.[61]

2. Contralateral AP, mortise, and lateral fluoroscopic views of the contralateral ankle are obtained for comparison of the operative syndesmosis reduction.

3. Medial malleolar fracture, if present, should be anatomically fixed first through a medial incision.

4. A 6- to 8-cm incision is made over the distal fibula through skin directly onto bone. Care should be made to protect the superficial peroneal nerve.

5. Appropriate retractors are placed to retract the peroneal tendons posteriorly to fully visualize the lateral malleolus fracture. Interposed periosteum is then resected from the fracture site.

6. A reduction maneuver is performed to reduce the lateral malleolus fracture anatomically and out to length. If the posterior malleolar fracture is large and displaced, it should be fixed before plate fixation of the fibula because the plate may obscure the lateral images of the tibial plafond. In addition, displaced fractures of the posterior malleolus can be facilitated by removal of interposed bony fragments from the approach through the lateral malleolar fracture.

7. Fixation of concomitant posterior malleolus is performed with percutaneous anterior to posterior screw or direct fixation with a posterior buttress plate or screws.
   a. Posterior malleolus fixation has been shown to improve syndesmosis stability.[74–77]

8. The lateral malleolus fracture is then fixed with a one-third tubular plate-and-screw construct to ensure adequate fixation above and below the fracture line. A lag screw may be placed if needed before plate fixation.
   a. In patients with length-stable Maisonneuve fractures, syndesmotic screw-only fixation can be used.

9. Appropriate placement of fixation and fibula length is confirmed on fluoroscopy.

10. Avulsion injuries of the AITFL (ie, Chaput or Wagstaff fragments) can be fixed with a screw-and-washer construct.

11. Assessment of syndesmosis stability is performed by AP and mortise fluoroscopic

imaging via the cotton hook test[78] or external rotation stress test with direct observation.

a. If significant widening of the distal tibiofibular joint occurs, syndesmotic fixation should be performed. Care should be taken to also assess sagittal syndesmotic instability on the lateral view.[18] The fibula normally rests in the incisura fibularis and should overlap the posterior one-third of the tibia. If the fibula can be displaced toward the anterior half of the tibia, syndesmotic fixation should be performed.

12. The previous lateral ankle incision is dissected anteriorly to directly visualize the anterior syndesmosis.

13. Steps 12 to 16 from the previous section are followed if syndesmosis fixation is needed.

Key Pitfalls

- If considerable force is required to restore the tibiofibular relation or if the medial clear space widening is present, consider performing a medial approach over the ankle to assess the deltoid ligament.

- In the pediatric population, inadequate syndesmosis reduction despite adequate reduction maneuver may indicate plastic deformity of the fibula. A proximal fibular osteotomy should be considered in these cases to prevent disruption of the interosseous ligament.[3]

POSTOPERATIVE CARE
Isolated Syndesmosis Fixation

- Weeks 0 to 2: non–weight bearing in a postoperative splint for 14 days until sutures are removed.
- Weeks 2 to 6: partial weight bearing with a walking boot. Patient may begin physical therapy to work on gentle ankle range of motion.
- Weeks 6 to 12: full weight bearing with shoes.
- 3 to 6 months: return to play.

Syndesmosis Fixation with Concomitant Fracture

- Weeks 0 to 2: non–weight bearing in a postoperative splint for 14 days until sutures are removed.

- Weeks 2 to 6: continue non–weight bearing in a boot. May work on ankle range of motion.
- Week 6 to 12: progressive weight bearing in shoes. May progress to strengthening
- Months 3 to 6: full weight bearing with shoes. Progressive return to baseline activities.

COMPLICATIONS AND MANAGEMENT

The complications after direct syndesmosis repair and reconstruction have not been well described in the literature. Given that direct repair is often supplemented with suture-button or screw constructs, complications associated with these procedures are listed in **Table 1.**

OUTCOMES

The literature suggests poor results with syndesmotic injuries in the setting of ankle sprains[26] and ankle fractures.[83–85] Burns and colleagues[20] showed that combined deltoid and syndesmosis disruption leads to 0.73-mm syndesmosis diastasis and 39% reduction of ankle contact area during axial loading. In addition, 1 mm of lateral talar translation within the ankle mortise can lead to a 43% reduction in total contact area of the ankle joint, potentially leading to arthritis.[86]

The quality of syndesmosis reduction seems to be the main factor for improving clinical outcomes after syndesmotic injuries.[9,37,43,63,84,85] However, plain radiographs are not accurate in detecting rotational syndesmosis malreduction.[53,54,87] Chissell and Jones[85] found that Weber type C ankle fracture with greater than 1.5 mm of syndesmosis diastasis on plain radiographs after screw fixation led to worse outcomes. Similarly, Miller and colleagues[43] showed that CT scan malreduction of the syndesmosis greater than 2 mm after direct visualization leads to worse outcomes. Leeds and Ehrlich[9] followed 34 patients with bimalleolar and trimalleolar fractures for 4 years and found that the inadequate lateral malleolus and syndesmosis reduction correlated with worse patient outcomes and arthritis. Weening and Bhandari[84] followed a cohort of 39 ankle fractures with syndesmosis injuries for 18 months and found that unreduced syndesmosis at the time of ankle fixation led to poorer Short Musculoskeletal Functional Assessment (SMFA) scores and Olerud-Molander scores compared with

Table 1
Complications associated with direct syndesmosis repair and reconstruction

Complication	Management	Comments
Syndesmosis malreduction[63]	Intraoperative: carefully assess lateral fluoroscopic images for sagittal malreduction. Redirect reduction clamps prior to definitive fixation. Postoperative: obtain weight-bearing CT scan to determine direction of malreduction and incisura fibularis morphology.[79,80] May perform revision fixation if needed	Sagi et al,[63] 2012: 27 of 68 malreductions (39%) on CT imaging
Suture-button knot prominene[40]	Cover fibular periosteal sleeve over the lateral knot at the time of wound closure	3 of 18 (16.7%) without periosteal sleeve 0 of 31 (0%) in modified technique
Suture-button construct loosening[41]	Avoid using limited-contact dynamic compression plates. Use 1/3 tubular plates to prevent toggling of the Suture-button from within the screw hole	Case series of 3 patients
Tendon entrapment[81]	Hardware removal	Avoid excessive anterior suture-button divergence if 2 constructs are used
Syndesmosis diastasis	Hardware removal	
Injury to perforating branch of peroneal artery[64]	Careful placement of superior fixation if 2 suture-button or screw constructs are used	Peroneal artery penetrates 3.42 cm proximal to tibial plafond
Symptomatic screw[31–33,82]	Screw removal at 6 mo	Screw removal of intact screws can improve ankle range of motion and clinical outcomes. Mild diastasis can be found after screw removal. There is no clear evidence that supports the routine removal of screws in asymptomatic patients
Screw breakage[83]	Surgical removal	18 of 144 (13%) at 1-year follow-up

individuals who underwent syndesmosis fixation. Sagi and colleagues[63] studied 107 patients with ankle fractures and concomitant syndesmosis injuries who underwent either open reduction or indirect reduction and screw fixation. The investigators found that 39% of patients had malreduction of the syndesmosis at a minimum of 2 years' follow-up, leading to worse SMFA and Olerund-Molander scores.

The resurgence of direct syndesmosis repair has attempted to address the shortcomings of syndesmosis screw fixation and suture-button constructs. Biomechanically, ligament repair has been shown to be as strong as syndesmosis screw fixation.[88] Goetz and colleagues[89] showed that anatomic syndesmosis repair was required to restore external rotation stability of the syndesmosis. The clinical outcomes specific to anatomic repair of the syndesmosis are outlined in **Table 2**.

Table 2
Clinical outcomes specific to anatomic repair of the syndesmosis

Authors, Ref. Year	Level of Evidence	Cohort/ Indication	Sample Size	Mean Age (y)	Follow-Up	Measurement Tools	Outcome	Complications
Kabukcuoglu et al,[90] 2000	IV	Supination-external rotation, pronation-external rotation (PER), and pronation-abduction (PAB) fractures undergoing ANK device fixation (fibula nail and tibial screw-post AITFL repair)	49	36.3	39 mo	Baird and Jackson	59.2% excellent, 24.5% good, 10.2% fair, 6.1% poor	Fibular malreduction (n = 4)
Grass et al,[91] 2003	IV	Chronic PER III/IV and PAB II syndesmosis injuries undergoing AITFL reconstruction using split peroneus longus tendon	16		16.4 y	Karlsson score and radiographic/CT scan follow-up	Improvement in medial radiographic reduction	0% infection, 7.1% screw failure, 7.1% synostosis, 7.1% dysesthesias
Nelson,[55] 2006	IV	Bimalleolar trimalleolar, and bimalleolar equivalent fixations undergoing open AITFL repair with screw-washer construct	50	48.8	6 mo	N/A	98% radiographic anatomic reduction on mortise view	10% persistent instability (n = 1) Hardware removal (HWR) for extensor hallucis longus irritation (n = 3), Hardware failure in a neuropathic patient (n = 1)
Little et al,[92] 2015	III-comparative	SER-IV fractures *Group 1 = PITFL repair (screw and washer) and deltoid repair (MiTek anchor) Group 2 = syndesmosis screw*	45	46	12 mo	Postoperative radiograph and CT scans	Similar ROM	*Group 1: malreduction 7.4%, major wound 3.7%, 11% HWR Group 2 = malreduction 33.3%, major wound 0%, HWR 78%*

(continued on next page)

Table 7
(continued)

Authors, Ref. Year	Level of Evidence	Cohort/ Indication	Sample Size	Mean Age (y)	Follow-Up	Measurement Tools	Outcome	Complications
Jones and Nunley,[93] 2015	III	SER-IV ankle fractures *Group 1 = syndesmosis screw and routine HWR* *Group 2 = deltoid repair with suture anchor*	27	35	50.25 mo	Lower extremity function Foot and Ankle Disability score, SMFA score, Foot and Ankle Outcome, American Orthopedic Foot and Ankle score, visual analog score of pain	No difference in outcome scores for either group	Group 1: malreduction 7%, wound dehiscence 7% Group 2: malreduction 0%
Hsu et al,[73] 2015	IV	NFL players with PER ankle fractures undergoing ankle arthroscopy, Tightrope syndesmosis fixation, and deltoid repair with suture anchor	14	25	21.6 mo	Return to play, games played	Return to play 6 mo (86%)	No evidence of ankle pain, increased medial clear space, or arthritis
Zhan et al,[94] 2016	IV-comparative	External rotation ankle fractures with posterior malleolus fracture fixation *Group 1 = AITFL repair* *Group 2 = syndesmosis screw*	53	44.5	12 mo	Olerud-Molander scores	No difference in outcomes for repair (90.4) vs screw (85.5) Return to work: AITFL repair 5.26 mo vs 7.15 mo	*AITFL repair:* Malreduction 7.4%, 0% infection *Screw fixation:* malreduction 19.2%, broken screws 11.5%, rediastasis 11.5%, 3.8% wound infection

SUMMARY

- The resurgence of direct syndesmosis repair has attempted to address the shortcomings of syndesmosis screw fixation and suture-button constructs.
- Biomechanically, anatomic ligament repair has been shown to be as strong as syndesmosis screw fixation.
- The quality of syndesmosis reduction seems to be the main factor for improving clinical outcomes after syndesmotic injuries.

REFERENCES

1. Mauntel TC, Wikstrom EA, Roos KG, et al. The epidemiology of high ankle sprains in National Collegiate Athletic Association Sports. Am J Sports Med 2017;45(9):2156–63.
2. Mulcahey MK, Bernhardson AS, Murphy CP, et al. The epidemiology of ankle injuries identified at the National Football League combine, 2009-2015. Orthop J Sports Med 2018;6(7). 2325967118786227.
3. Edwards GS Jr, DeLee JC. Ankle diastasis without fracture. Foot Ankle 1984;4(6):305–12.
4. Dattani R, Patnaik S, Kantak A, et al. Injuries to the tibiofibular syndesmosis. J Bone Joint Surg Br 2008;90(4):405–10.
5. Pankovich AM. Maisonneuve fracture of the fibula. J Bone Joint Surg Am 1976;58(3):337–42.
6. maisonneuve J. Recherches sur la fracture du perone. Arch Gen Med 1840;7:165.
7. Mason LW, Marlow WJ, Widnall J, et al. Pathoanatomy and associated injuries of posterior malleolus fracture of the ankle. Foot Ankle Int 2017;38(11):1229–35.
8. Carr JC 2nd, Werner BC, Yarboro SR. An update on management of syndesmosis injury: a national US database study. Am J Orthop (Belle Mead NJ) 2016;45(7):E472–e477.
9. Leeds HC, Ehrlich MG. Instability of the distal tibiofibular syndesmosis after bimalleolar and trimalleolar ankle fractures. J Bone Joint Surg Am 1984;66(4):490–503.
10. Sarrafian S. Osteology. In: Kelikian AS, Sarrafian SK, editors. Anatomy of the foot and ankle: descriptive, topographic, functional. 2nd edition. Philadelphia: J.B. Lippincott Company; 1993. p. 37–58.
11. Hermans JJ, Beumer A, de Jong TA, et al. Anatomy of the distal tibiofibular syndesmosis in adults: a pictorial essay with a multimodality approach. J Anat 2010;217(6):633–45.
12. Walling A, Sanders R, Behboudi A, et al. Ankle fractures. In: Coughlin MJ, Saltzman CL, Anderson RB, editors. Mann's surgery of the foot and ankle. 9th edition. Philadelphia: Elsevier; 2014. p. 2003–40.
13. Lilyquist M, Shaw A, Latz K, et al. Cadaveric analysis of the distal tibiofibular syndesmosis. Foot Ankle Int 2016;37(8):882–90.
14. Williams BT, Ahrberg AB, Goldsmith MT, et al. Ankle syndesmosis: a qualitative and quantitative anatomic analysis. Am J Sports Med 2015;43(1):88–97.
15. Campbell KJ, Michalski MP, Wilson KJ, et al. The ligament anatomy of the deltoid complex of the ankle: a qualitative and quantitative anatomical study. J Bone Joint Surg Am 2014;96(8):e62.
16. Clanton TO, Williams BT, Backus JD, et al. Biomechanical analysis of the individual ligament contributions to syndesmotic stability. Foot Ankle Int 2017;38(1):66–75.
17. Ogilvie-Harris DJ, Reed SC, Hedman TP. Disruption of the ankle syndesmosis: biomechanical study of the ligamentous restraints. Arthroscopy 1994;10(5):558–60.
18. Xenos JS, Hopkinson WJ, Mulligan ME, et al. The tibiofibular syndesmosis. Evaluation of the ligamentous structures, methods of fixation, and radiographic assessment. J Bone Joint Surg Am 1995;77(6):847–56.
19. Rasmussen O. Stability of the ankle joint. Analysis of the function and traumatology of the ankle ligaments. Acta Orthop Scand Suppl 1985;211:1–75.
20. Burns WC 2nd, Prakash K, Adelaar R, et al. Tibiotalar joint dynamics: indications for the syndesmotic screw—a cadaver study. Foot Ankle 1993;14(3):153–8.
21. Attarian DE, McCrackin HJ, DeVito DP, et al. Biomechanical characteristics of human ankle ligaments. Foot Ankle 1985;6(2):54–8.
22. Harper MC. Deltoid ligament: an anatomical evaluation of function. Foot Ankle 1987;8(1):19–22.
23. Earll M, Wayne J, Brodrick C, et al. Contribution of the deltoid ligament to ankle joint contact characteristics: a cadaver study. Foot Ankle Int 1996;17(6):317–24.
24. Hunt KJ, Phisitkul P, Pirolo J, et al. High ankle sprains and syndesmotic injuries in athletes. J Am Acad Orthop Surg 2015;23(11):661–73.
25. Takao M, Ochi M, Oae K, et al. Diagnosis of a tear of the tibiofibular syndesmosis. The role of arthroscopy of the ankle. J Bone Joint Surg Br 2003;85(3):324–9.
26. Sikka RS, Fetzer GB, Sugarman E, et al. Correlating MRI findings with disability in syndesmotic sprains of NFL players. Foot Ankle Int 2012;33(5):371–8.
27. Feller R, Borenstein T, Fantry AJ, et al. Arthroscopic quantification of syndesmotic instability in a cadaveric model. Arthroscopy 2017;33(2):436–44.
28. Lui TH, Ip K, Chow HT. Comparison of radiologic and arthroscopic diagnoses of distal tibiofibular syndesmosis disruption in acute ankle fracture. Arthroscopy 2005;21(11):1370.

29. Andersen MR, Frihagen F, Madsen JE, et al. High complication rate after syndesmotic screw removal. Injury 2015;46(11):2283–7.

30. Schepers T, Van Lieshout EM, de Vries MR, et al. Complications of syndesmotic screw removal. Foot Ankle Int 2011;32(11):1040–4.

31. Miller AN, Paul O, Boraiah S, et al. Functional outcomes after syndesmotic screw fixation and removal. J Orthop Trauma 2010;24(1):12–6.

32. Dingemans SA, Rammelt S, White TO, et al. Should syndesmotic screws be removed after surgical fixation of unstable ankle fractures? a systematic review. Bone Joint J 2016;98-B(11):1497–504.

33. Gennis E, Koenig S, Rodericks D, et al. The fate of the fixed syndesmosis over time. Foot Ankle Int 2015;36(10):1202–8.

34. LaMothe JM, Baxter JR, Murphy C, et al. Three-dimensional analysis of fibular motion after fixation of syndesmotic injuries with a screw or suture-button construct. Foot Ankle Int 2016;37(12):1350–6.

35. Westermann RW, Rungprai C, Goetz JE, et al. The effect of suture-button fixation on simulated syndesmotic malreduction: a cadaveric study. J Bone Joint Surg Am 2014;96(20):1732–8.

36. Thornes B, Shannon F, Guiney AM, et al. Suture-button syndesmosis fixation: accelerated rehabilitation and improved outcomes. Clin Orthop Relat Res 2005;(431):207–12.

37. Naqvi GA, Cunningham P, Lynch B, et al. Fixation of ankle syndesmotic injuries: comparison of tightrope fixation and syndesmotic screw fixation for accuracy of syndesmotic reduction. Am J Sports Med 2012;40(12):2828–35.

38. Clanton TO, Whitlow SR, Williams BT, et al. Biomechanical comparison of 3 current ankle syndesmosis repair techniques. Foot Ankle Int 2017; 38(2):200–7.

39. Schon JM, Williams BT, Venderley MB, et al. A 3-D CT analysis of screw and suture-button fixation of the syndesmosis. Foot Ankle Int 2017;38(2):208–14.

40. Naqvi GA, Shafqat A, Awan N. Tightrope fixation of ankle syndesmosis injuries: clinical outcome, complications and technique modification. Injury 2012; 43(6):838–42.

41. Ibnu Samsudin M, Yap MQW, Wei Luong A, et al. Slippage of tightrope button in syndesmotic fixation of Weber C Malleolar fractures: a case series. Foot Ankle Int 2018;39(5):613–7.

42. Willmott HJ, Singh B, David LA. Outcome and complications of treatment of ankle diastasis with tightrope fixation. Injury 2009;40(11):1204–6.

43. Miller AN, Carroll EA, Parker RJ, et al. Direct visualization for syndesmotic stabilization of ankle fractures. Foot Ankle Int 2009;30(5):419–26.

44. Guyton GP, DeFontes K 3rd, Barr CR, et al. Arthroscopic correlates of subtle syndesmotic injury. Foot Ankle Int 2017;38(5):502–6.

45. Nussbaum ED, Hosea TM, Sieler SD, et al. Prospective evaluation of syndesmotic ankle sprains without diastasis. Am J Sports Med 2001;29(1):31–5.

46. Sman AD, Hiller CE, Rae K, et al. Diagnostic accuracy of clinical tests for ankle syndesmosis injury. Br J Sports Med 2015;49(5):323–9.

47. Calder JD, Bamford R, Petrie A, et al. Stable versus unstable grade II high ankle sprains: a prospective study predicting the need for surgical stabilization and time to return to sports. Arthroscopy 2016; 32(4):634–42.

48. McConnell T, Creevy W, Tornetta P 3rd. Stress examination of supination external rotation-type fibular fractures. J Bone Joint Surg Am 2004;86-A(10):2171–8.

49. Giordano CP, Koval KJ, Zuckerman JD, et al. Fracture blisters. Clin Orthop Relat Res 1994;(307): 214–21.

50. Strauss EJ, Petrucelli G, Bong M, et al. Blisters associated with lower-extremity fracture: results of a prospective treatment protocol. J Orthop Trauma 2006;20(9):618–22.

51. White TO, Bugler KE, Appleton P, et al. A prospective randomised controlled trial of the fibular nail versus standard open reduction and internal fixation for fixation of ankle fractures in elderly patients. Bone Joint J 2016;98-B(9):1248–52.

52. Ashman BD, Kong C, Wing KJ, et al. Fluoroscopy-guided reduction and fibular nail fixation to manage unstable ankle fractures in patients with diabetes: a retrospective cohort study. Bone Joint J 2016;98-B(9):1197–201.

53. Ebraheim NA, Lu J, Yang H, et al. Radiographic and CT evaluation of tibiofibular syndesmotic diastasis: a cadaver study. Foot Ankle Int 1997;18(11):693–8.

54. Beumer A, van Hemert WL, Niesing R, et al. Radiographic measurement of the distal tibiofibular syndesmosis has limited use. Clin Orthop Relat Res 2004;(423):227–34.

55. Nelson OA. Examination and repair of the AITFL in transmalleolar fractures. J Orthop Trauma 2006; 20(9):637–43.

56. Boden SD, Labropoulos PA, McCowin P, et al. Mechanical considerations for the syndesmosis screw. A cadaver study. J Bone Joint Surg Am 1989;71(10): 1548–55.

57. Nielson JH, Sallis JG, Potter HG, et al. Correlation of interosseous membrane tears to the level of the fibular fracture. J Orthop Trauma 2004;18(2): 68–74.

58. Dikos GD, Heisler J, Choplin RH, et al. Normal tibiofibular relationships at the syndesmosis on axial CT imaging. J Orthop Trauma 2012;26(7): 433–8.

59. Nault ML, Hebert-Davies J, Laflamme GY, et al. CT scan assessment of the syndesmosis: a new

reproducible method. J Orthop Trauma 2013; 27(11):638–41.

60. Ahn TK, Choi SM, Kim JY, et al. Isolated syndesmosis diastasis: computed tomography scan assessment with arthroscopic correlation. Arthroscopy 2017;33(4):828–34.

61. Tornetta P 3rd, Ricci W, Nork S, et al. The posterolateral approach to the tibia for displaced posterior malleolar injuries. J Orthop Trauma 2011;25(2): 123–6.

62. Michelson JD, Wright M, Blankstein M. Syndesmotic ankle fractures. J Orthop Trauma 2018; 32(1):10–4.

63. Sagi HC, Shah AR, Sanders RW. The functional consequence of syndesmotic joint malreduction at a minimum 2-year follow-up. J Orthop Trauma 2012;26(7):439–43.

64. Penera K, Manji K, Wedel M, et al. Ankle syndesmotic fixation using two screws: risk of injury to the perforating branch of the peroneal artery. J Foot Ankle Surg 2014;53(5):534–8.

65. McKeon KE, Wright RW, Johnson JE, et al. Vascular anatomy of the tibiofibular syndesmosis. J Bone Joint Surg Am 2012;94(10):931–8.

66. Tornetta P 3rd, Spoo JE, Reynolds FA, et al. Overtightening of the ankle syndesmosis: is it really possible? J Bone Joint Surg Am 2001;83-A(4): 489–92.

67. Pallis MP, Pressman DN, Heida K, et al. Effect of ankle position on tibiotalar motion with screw fixation of the distal tibiofibular syndesmosis in a fracture model. Foot Ankle Int 2018;39(6):746–50.

68. Gonzalez T, Egan J, Ghorbanhoseini M, et al. Overtightening of the syndesmosis revisited and the effect of syndesmotic malreduction on ankle dorsiflexion. Injury 2017;48(6):1253–7.

69. Phisitkul P, Ebinger T, Goetz J, et al. Forceps reduction of the syndesmosis in rotational ankle fractures: a cadaveric study. J Bone Joint Surg Am 2012;94(24):2256–61.

70. Cosgrove CT, Putnam SM, Cherney SM, et al. Medial clamp tine positioning affects ankle syndesmosis malreduction. J Orthop Trauma 2017;31(8): 440–6.

71. Lack W, Phisitkul P, Femino JE. Anatomic deltoid ligament repair with anchor-to-post suture reinforcement: technique tip. Iowa Orthop J 2012;32: 227–30.

72. Lee SH, Kim ES, Lee YK, et al. Arthroscopic syndesmotic repair: technical tip. Foot Ankle Int 2015; 36(2):229–31.

73. Hsu AR, Lareau CR, Anderson RB. Repair of acute superficial deltoid complex avulsion during ankle fracture fixation in national football league players. Foot Ankle Int 2015;36(11):1272–8.

74. Gardner MJ, Brodsky A, Briggs SM, et al. Fixation of posterior malleolar fractures provides greater

syndesmotic stability. Clin Orthop Relat Res 2006; 447:165–71.

75. Miller AN, Carroll EA, Parker RJ, et al. Posterior malleolar stabilization of syndesmotic injuries is equivalent to screw fixation. Clin Orthop Relat Res 2010;468(4):1129–35.

76. Miller MA, McDonald TC, Graves ML, et al. Stability of the syndesmosis after posterior malleolar fracture fixation. Foot Ankle Int 2018;39(1): 99–104.

77. Fitzpatrick E, Goetz JE, Sittapairoj T, et al. Effect of posterior malleolus fracture on syndesmotic reduction: a cadaveric study. J Bone Joint Surg Am 2018; 100(3):243–8.

78. Cotton F. Fractures and joint dislocations. Philadelphia: WB Saunders; 1910.

79. Cherney SM, Spraggs-Hughes AG, McAndrew CM, et al. Incisura morphology as a risk factor for syndesmotic malreduction. Foot Ankle Int 2016;37(7): 748–54.

80. Boszczyk A, Kwapisz S, Krummel M, et al. Correlation of incisura anatomy with syndesmotic malreduction. Foot Ankle Int 2018;39(3):369–75.

81. Welck MJ, Ray P. Tibialis anterior tendon entrapment after ankle tightrope insertion for acute syndesmosis injury. Foot Ankle Spec 2013;6(3):242–6.

82. Manjoo A, Sanders DW, Tieszer C, et al. Functional and radiographic results of patients with syndesmotic screw fixation: implications for screw removal. J Orthop Trauma 2010;24(1):2–6.

83. Egol KA, Pahk B, Walsh M, et al. Outcome after unstable ankle fracture: effect of syndesmotic stabilization. J Orthop Trauma 2010;24(1):7–11.

84. Weening B, Bhandari M. Predictors of functional outcome following transsyndesmotic screw fixation of ankle fractures. J Orthop Trauma 2005;19(2): 102–8.

85. Chissell HR, Jones J. The influence of a diastasis screw on the outcome of Weber type-C ankle fractures. J Bone Joint Surg Br 1995;77(3):435–8.

86. Ramsey PL, Hamilton W. Changes in tibiotalar area of contact caused by lateral talar shift. J Bone Joint Surg Am 1976;58(3):356–7.

87. Gardner MJ, Demetrakopoulos D, Briggs SM, et al. Malreduction of the tibiofibular syndesmosis in ankle fractures. Foot Ankle Int 2006;27(10): 788–92.

88. Schottel PC, Baxter J, Gilbert S, et al. Anatomic ligament repair restores ankle and syndesmotic rotational stability as much as syndesmotic screw fixation. J Orthop Trauma 2016;30(2):e36–40.

89. Goetz JE, Davidson NP, Rudert MJ, et al. Biomechanical comparison of syndesmotic repair techniques during external rotation stress. Foot Ankle Int 2018;39(11):1345–54.

90. Kabukcuoglu Y, Kucukkaya M, Eren T, et al. The ANK device: a new approach in the treatment of

the fractures of the lateral malleolus associated with the rupture of the syndesmosis. Foot Ankle Int 2000;21(9):753–8.

91. Grass R, Rammelt S, Biewener A, et al. Peroneus longus ligamentoplasty for chronic instability of the distal tibiofibular syndesmosis. Foot Ankle Int 2003;24(5):392–7.

92. Little MM, Berkes MB, Schottel PC, et al. Anatomic fixation of supination external rotation type IV equivalent ankle fractures. J Orthop Trauma 2015; 29(5):250–5.

93. Jones CR, Nunley JA 2nd. Deltoid ligament repair versus syndesmotic fixation in bimalleolar equivalent ankle fractures. J Orthop Trauma 2015;29(5): 245–9.

94. Zhan Y, Yan X, Xia R, et al. Anterior-inferior tibiofibular ligament anatomical repair and augmentation versus trans-syndesmosis screw fixation for the syndesmotic instability in external-rotation type ankle fracture with posterior malleolus involvement: A prospective and comparative study. Injury 2016;47(7):1574–80.

Printed and bound by CPI Group (UK) Ltd, Croydon, CR0 4YY

08/05/2025

01864745-0019